Locked in the Family Cell

Irish Studies in Literature and Culture

MICHAEL PATRICK GILLESPIE

SERIES EDITOR

Locked in the Family Cell

Gender, Sexuality, and
Political Agency in Irish
National Discourse

Kathryn A. Conrad

THE UNIVERSITY OF WISCONSIN PRESS

The University of Wisconsin Press
1930 Monroe Street
Madison, Wisconsin 53711

www.wisc.edu/wisconsinpress/

3 Henrietta Street
London WC2E 8LU, England

5   4   3   2   1

Library of Congress Cataloging-in-Publication Data
Conrad, Kathryn A.
Locked in the family cell : gender, sexuality, and political agency in Irish national
discourse / Kathryn A. Conrad.
    p. cm. — (Irish studies in literature and culture)
    Includes bibliographical references and index.
    ISBN 0-299-19650-X (cloth : alk. paper)
    1. Family—Political aspects—Ireland. 2. Sexual orientation—Political aspects—
Ireland. 3. Human reproduction—Social aspects—Ireland. 4. Social control—Ireland.
5. Sex role—Ireland.
I. Title. II. Series.
HQ620.C65   2004
306.85'09415—dc22   2003020573

In memory of
M. Elizabeth Conrad
W. Arthur Conrad
J. Bernard VanderMeer

Contents

Illustrations

Acknowledgments

The network of colleagues, relatives, and friends who have supported me through this project is my own best example of the positive force of family, broadly defined.

This book has gone through several stages, the first of which being its life as my dissertation at the University of Pennsylvania. My adviser, Vicki Mahaffey, was my greatest influence and inspiration both prior to and during that process. Through her I also gained a lasting appreciation of James Joyce, who, while he does not appear in this book, has nonetheless greatly affected the way I think about language and power. I am also indebted to my dissertation readers, Inés Salazar, Roger Abrahams, and Jean-Michel Rabaté; my dissertation support group, Darryl Wadsworth and Allen Grove; and my many friends in the English and Comparative Literature Departments, especially Marian Eide and Nicholas Miller, for their input and support during my time at Penn and beyond.

As the project moved into its current form, innumerable colleagues and friends helped me to shape and polish my ideas. During my research in the Republic and the North, I was introduced to a network of scholars, artists, archivists, and activists whose input shaped my thinking on this project. In Dublin, Ailbhe Smyth and Katherine O'Donnell showed particular generosity of mind and spirit and provided the contacts that helped take the project in a new direction. The women of the Downtown Women's Centre, particularly Marie Mulholland, and the members of QueerSpace made my 1998 trip to Belfast far more pleasant and productive that I thought possible. Yvonne Murphy and Ciaran Crossey at the Linen Hall Library's Northern Ireland Political Collection have been essential to my research, most notably during my long visit in 2000; their help, dedication, and ability to define Northern Ireland politics more broadly than most has enriched this project beyond measure. Filmmaker Margo Harkin opened her archives and her home to me, and I remain grateful for her generosity and continued friendship. Closer to home, New York's ILGO founders Anne Maguire and Marie Honan have provided me not only with insights, challenges, and connections, but also with friendship and inspiration.

Some of the best feedback I received on the work in progress came from members of the American Conference for Irish Studies, who have heard segments of this book over the last few years at international and regional conferences. The officers of the ACIS deserve thanks for encouraging younger scholars and progressive approaches to Irish studies. I also appreciate the invitations to present my work at the University of Illinois at Urbana-Champaign and the University of Houston; the feedback those lectures generated has been invaluable, and the hospitality I received was unparalleled. My own university, the University of Kansas, has provided me with several opportunities to present my work in the Hall Center for the Humanities Gender and Nationalism, Migration and Displacement, and Gender seminars for faculty; I particularly appreciate the chairs of these seminars for providing the guiding force behind these valuable interdisciplinary exchanges and the Hall Center staff and leadership for making them possible. My compatriots in the Gender and Nationalism seminar—Omofolabo Ajayi, Lorraine Bayard de Volo, Bart Dean, Misty Gerner, Gwynne Jenkins, Michelle McKinley, Joane Nagel, Judith Richards, and Lee Skinner—all deserve special thanks for making interdisciplinary inquiry not only productive but fun.

In these and other forums, many have offered insights, close readings of my work, advice, and encouragement. Giselle Anatol, Lisa Bitel, Byron Caminero-Santangelo, Marta Caminero-Santangelo, Gregory Castle, Julie Crawford, Elizabeth Cullingford, Dorice Elliott, Adrian Frazier, Richard Haslam, Susan Cannon Harris, Mary Klayder, Colleen Lamos, Cheryl Lester, Ed Madden, Peter McAuley, Anna Neill, Rhiannon Talbot, Spurgeon Thompson, Joseph Valente, Amanda Yeates, Liza Yukins, and Heather Zwicker have all helped to sustain me intellectually during this process. Teaching, of course, has helped me shape my ideas, and I owe a debt of gratitude to those students who have been part of that process, particularly in my Irish literature and culture classes. My chairs in the Department of English—James Hartman, Richard Hardin, and Bernard Hirsch—have been instrumental in promoting a collegial environment and have been wonderfully supportive during even the most difficult times. At the University of Wisconsin Press, I am particularly indebted to Michael Gillespie, the Irish Literature and Culture Series editor, for his enthusiasm about the project and his guidance of this novice through the many stages of publication; and Tricia Brock, who has helped immeasurably with the important details. And although they bear no responsibility for the weaknesses of this text, Nancy Curtin and Margot Backus — thanks to their careful and insightful readings of this manuscript, their advice and encouragement during the writing process, and their own example as outstanding scholars whom I can only hope to emulate — deserve much of the credit for its strengths.

Finally, without the support and love of members of my chosen family, I could not have completed this project. My love and gratitude to Joan, Boyd, Paul, Julie, Alex, and Austin Conrad; Gayle VanderMeer; Heidi and Charlie Vonk; Darryl Wadsworth; Phil, Retha, and Kevin Willis; Chelsea Cantwell; and Kory Willis, who has taught me the meaning of joy and given my life balance.

This project received funding from several sources. While at the University of Pennsylvania, I benefited from financial support from the Graduate School and the Department of English as well as the Woodrow Wilson Foundation's Mellon Fellowships in the Humanities. Since coming to the University of Kansas, I have been grateful for the support from the Department of English, the Center for Research, Inc., and the Hall Center for the Humanities.

Although they have been much revised, portions of this book have appeared in the following published essays: "Fetal Ireland: National Bodies and Political Agency," *Éire-Ireland: An Interdisciplinary Journal of Irish Studies* 36.3–4 (Fall/Winter 2001): 153–73; "Queer Treasons: Homosexuality and Irish National Identity," *Cultural Studies* 15.1 (January 2001): 124–37 (archived at http://www.tandf.co.uk [subscription only]); "Women Troubles, Queer Troubles: Gender, Sexuality, and the Politics of Selfhood in the Construction of the Northern Irish State," in *Reclaiming Gender: Transgressive Identities in Modern Ireland*, ed. Marilyn Cohen and Nancy Curtin, 53–67 (New York: St. Martin's Press, 1999); "Occupied Country: The Negotiation of Lesbianism in Irish Feminist Writing," *Éire-Ireland: An Interdisciplinary Journal of Irish Studies* 31.1–2 (Spring/Summer 1996): 123–36. My thanks to the publishers of these articles for permission to include portions of those articles here.

Thanks also to Margo Harkin, for permission to reproduce film stills from *Hush-A-Bye Baby*, and to Martyn Turner, for permission to reproduce the X-Case cartoon. Full credits appear in the captions to those illustrations.

Locked in the Family Cell

Introduction
Informing on the Irish Family Cell

Cell: from the Indo-European root kel, to cover or conceal.

I really believe that the pagans, and the abortionists, and the feminists, and the gays and the lesbians who are actively trying to make that an alternative lifestyle, the ACLU, People for the American Way—all of them who have tried to secularize America—I point the finger in their face and say, "You helped this happen."
—Rev. Jerry Falwell, after the September 11, 2001, attacks on the World Trade Center and Pentagon in the United States

The place of Ireland in the new Europe, the troubles in the North, women's and gay rights campaigns in the North and South: all provide points of entry into this project. I have chosen to begin, however, with a comment by an American fundamentalist Christian, Reverend Jerry Falwell, speaking after the September 11, 2001, attacks on the United States. Falwell's comments not only speak to the prevalence of the attitudes I treat in *Locked in the Family Cell* but also suggest the urgency with which they must be addressed.

Falwell represents an extreme, but the ideology he reinforces in this statement is far more mainstream than it first appears and is not, I suggest, founded solely in Christian religious discourse *or* confined to the United States. His statement suggests that the threat "over there" is dependent upon a threat "here"—a threat to family and by extension a threat to the nation. He shares with many the belief that maintaining and containing the heterosexual family is thus the most effective way to

3

control borders, to reproduce the nation and state, to ensure "stability," and thus to prevent further terror.[1] But such a view, as I argue through-out the book, only freezes the public sphere and reentrenches a limiting discourse of containment and exclusion. The effects are most obviously felt by those who do not fit the model and are excluded, silenced, or pun-ished; but all, even those who seem empowered within the system, are held hostage by it, trapped within the family cell. This state of affairs means political stagnation, the death of a public sphere, and justification for continued abuses of power — all in the name of the family.

The Family Cell as Survival: A Brief History

The prison cell, the monastic cell, the biological cell, the revolutionary cell: each of these terms has in common enclosure and containment. Michel Foucault adds another to the list: the family cell. In *The History of Sexuality*, Foucault describes the family cell as the form that, in eigh-teenth-century Europe, "made it possible for the main elements of the deployment of sexuality (the feminine body, infantile precocity, the reg-ulation of births, and to a lesser extent no doubt, the specification of the perverted) to develop along its two primary dimensions: the husband-wife axis and the parents-children axis."[2] The family cell, in other words, shapes both normative heterosexuality and that which falls outside of it. But more than this, I argue: the centrality of the family cell to social, eco-nomic, and political organization defines and limits not only acceptable sexuality but also the contours of the private sphere, the public sphere, and the nation itself.

In her description of the history of the family cell in Ireland, Margot Backus draws on Foucault's evocation of the term, although she locates the entrenchment of the family cell earlier than Foucault does.[3] The cap-italist family cell, Backus argues, is the core of European social struc-tures. The Irish focus on the nuclear family has often been treated as a phenomenon arising out of Catholic ideology, but it is important to note that this form, as Backus has so eloquently shown in her study of Anglo-Irish gothic fiction, cut across class and religious boundaries. Following Mary Condron (*The Serpent and the Goddess*), she suggests that gender and status distinctions, reinforced and stabilized in the late sixteenth and early seventeenth centuries during the rise of British settlement and control of Ireland, were already in process in medieval Ireland, thanks to the rise of a patriarchal Christianity; later English settlement and the strict order and penalization imposed by British law only hastened the process of consolidation. In other words, the dual forces of Christianity, which reinforced a patriarchal system of familial relationships, and British colonialism, which divided the land and penalized social formations that did not further British interests, helped to fix the heterosexual nuclear family as the primary unit group of Irish society. As Backus notes, women who did not fit the prescribed social roles bore the brunt of regulatory practices and punishments: "while early modern authorities embraced the nuclear family as an indispensable means for maintaining stability in a rapidly altering world, a spate of emerging laws, regulations, and social attitudes and practices fueled what [Christina] Larner has called a mass criminalization of women between 1550 and 1700" for a variety of activities, from practicing witchcraft to committing infanticide to keeping house poorly (Backus, 37). But men, too, found punishment for transgressing the family cell: sodomy, "that utterly confused category" (Foucault, 101), was punishable by death from 1553, and death by fire, according to Foucault, was practiced until well into the eighteenth century. As Jonathan Goldberg has argued, sodomy, defined in practice as "any sexual act . . . that does not promote the aim of married procreative sex," only "emerges into visibility when those who are said to have done [it] also can be called traitors, heretics, or the like, at the very least, disturbers of the social order that alliance—marriage arrangements—maintained."[4]

As capital increasingly became the center of the economic universe, the domestic family cell became a necessity for economic as well as social survival for Catholic and Protestant alike. As capitalism took hold as the primary economic system in Europe, the centralization of the family was further reinforced:

> Over the course of early modernity, Europe annihilated within itself a broad range of subjectivities through the destruction of individual subjects who were, regardless of their actual proclivities, made to represent forbidden subject positions. The newly enforced heterosexual, monogamous, childbearing dyad was pushed to the center of the social order as all available alternatives to it were symbolically destroyed, legislated against, or, later, representationally made to disappear. In order not to disappear themselves, those early modern adults that survived rapidly organized themselves into the sole sanctioned social unit: the capitalist family cell. . . . During this period, kinship bonds and community bonds in general atrophied. Needless to say, this was hardest on the poor and socially disenfranchised. . . . As more affluent members of society became less dependent on

> family connections for prestige and promotion and the poor be-
> came dependent on wages, rich and poor alike grew increasingly
> anxious to concentrate resources within the most narrowly de-
> fined family unit possible. In such an environment, ties of famil-
> ial or neighborly obligation that ranged beyond the nuclear
> family's narrow confines grew increasingly risky and unsustain-
> able. (Backus, 41–42)

Those who challenged the social order were, as Backus suggests, criminalized, exterminated, or contained within the family cell (41).

This pattern of contraction of the family cell can be seen in Ireland
particularly in the nineteenth century. Women in rural households were
generally an essential part of the family economy, as was the case, for example, in the large number of families involved in the linen industry.[5]
The wages brought in to the family, facilitated by "the under- and often
unremunerated labor of women" (Gray, 44), encouraged the expansion
of household size as families took on income-producing members.[6] Such
conditions encouraged the subdivision of land holdings, early marriage,
and population growth. But the large family was not easily sustainable,
particularly after the arrival first of the mill-based spinning industry, which further suppressed wages for household spinners and
weavers, and then the potato blight, which pushed most subsistence-
level households beyond their capacity for survival.

Throughout the nineteenth century, many Irish women did move
into industrial work, particularly in the mill industries. But as those
women moved out of the home, they found themselves still shaped by
public discourse about a woman's place and value and still thus ultimately dependent on the family cell. Even in the poorhouses, as Marilyn Cohen has noted, "the Poor Law accorded greater recognition to the
hardship of men," even as the Poor Law guardians still required of
women "the most onerous of labor services", since Victorian constructions of gender saw the male as inevitably the family breadwinner,
whether or not this was actually the case ("Ethnography," 122–23).

As Ellen Jordan has suggested, these assumptions were based in a
shift in the nineteenth-century view of gender; Britain saw the transition
from a primarily hierarchical view of gender (man over woman) to a
separate-spheres ideology in which "men and women's spheres were
increasingly regarded as one of opposition, of mutual exclusion."[7]
Women's place was in the private sphere, still under the guidance of the
male head of the household. Regardless of their class position, women
in the public sphere were thus subject to more scrutiny than men, par-

ticularly if their actions were seen in any way to undermine the family (45–46).

This separate-spheres ideology was intimately tied to a citizenship discourse that had shifted to accommodate a middle-class notion of masculinity, as Anna Clark has argued.[8] This new construction of masculinity responded to the accusations that commerce made men effeminate through luxury, instead stressing the "middle-class man's status as head of household [to counter] any suspicion of femininity" and the development of a "new 'public sphere' of associations" (266). Such ideology served to encourage the reproduction of the family cell. Men were expected to control the family cell and moderate the relationship between the private and public spheres. But this in turn arguably impacted male sexual expression: male homosexuality was seen to threaten not only the reproduction of bodies but the system of alliances between men, providing affective bonds and allegiances that might undermine both the family cell and the public sphere.

The social controls exercised upon sexuality were given further discursive support as the nineteenth century saw the rise of psychological discourse that described inappropriate female behaviors as "hysteria." As Foucault writes, women's bodies were generally "hystericized," "a threefold process whereby the feminine body was analyzed—qualified and disqualified—as being thoroughly saturated with sexuality; whereby it was integrated into the sphere of medical practices; whereby, finally, it was placed in organic communication with the social body (whose regulated fecundity it was supposed to ensure), the family space (of which it had to be a substantial and functional element), and the life of children (which it produced and had to guarantee, by virtue of a biologico-moral responsibility lasting through the entire period of the children's education)" (104). Whether one accepts the order of Foucault's formulation, it is clear that the medicalization of women's bodies built upon the discursive schism between the natural and the social, as Backus describes it (39), and pathologized as disorderly those who did not fit their prescribed roles as reproducers and caretakers of the family. At the same time, medico-psychological discourse was giving further support to the exclusion of "sodomites" by defining as "perversion" anything that did not fit the model of the heterosexual family (Foucault, 110–11).

The nascent discipline of evolutionary science in the nineteenth century transferred the so-called pathologies of individuals onto whole "races" of people, characterizing the Irish and other colonized people as disorderly and unstable. British and, later, American political cartoons represented the Irish as animalistic and apelike creatures; scientific theorists similarly focused on the faults of the Irish skull, comparing it to that of lower primates and those human groups seen as lower on the evolutionary ladder.[9] It is important to stress that this discourse was primarily, but not exclusively, applied to Irish Catholics; when Protestants stepped out of line, the same language could be used to categorize them, usually framed in terms of degeneration and corruption due to exposure to the Celt.

This "scientific" discourse is reflected in the political discourse of the era. C. L. Innes quotes Benjamin Disraeli in a letter to the *Times* in 1868: "[The Irish] hate our order, our civilization, our enterprising industry, our sustained courage, our decorous liberty, our pure religion. This wild, reckless, indolent, uncertain and superstitious race have no sympathy with the English character."[10] Even Matthew Arnold, arguably one of those who inspired the Irish literary renaissance of the late nineteenth and early twentieth centuries, echoes Disraeli: "Sentimental—*always ready to react against the despotism of fact*; that is the description a great friend of the Celt [Henri Martin] gives him; and it is not a bad description of the sentimental temperament. . . . Even in the world of spiritual creation, he has never, in spite of his admirable gifts of quick perception and warm emotion, succeeded perfectly, because he never has had steadiness, patience, sanity enough to comply with the conditions under which alone can expression be perfectly given to the finest perceptions and emotions."[11] Arnold further characterized the Irish Celt as a feminine race (82), a discursive strategy not uncommon in imperial discourse and present in English descriptions of the Irish from at least as early as Spenser.[12] Women, like the children and animals to which the Irish were often compared, were below (civilized) men in the social order; the feminine Irish thus needed proper, orderly, masculine control. The trope of the "national family" projected the gendered domestic hierarchy—man over woman—onto affairs of nation and state by suggesting that the nation was, as Nira Yuval-Davis has put it, a "natural extension of family and kinship relations . . . . in which the men protect the 'womanandchildren.'"[13] Anne McClintock has further argued that "the family offered an indispensable trope for figuring what was often violent, *historical* change as natural, *organic* time. Since children 'naturally' progress into adults, projecting the family image on to national and imperial 'Progress' enabled what was often murderously violent change to be legitimized as the progressive unfolding of natural decree."[14] Reinforcing these constructions, Britain's answer to the Irish problem in particular lay in the political trope of marriage, as Innes suggests; Britain, the paternal John Bull, should rescue the maiden Hibernia and restore order, both to Irish culture and to the disorderly Irish political situation (14–15).

"Scientific" discourse thus only further entrenched the family cell as the foundational unit of Irish society, working in concert with the discourses of capitalism, religion, and the British state. By the end of the nineteenth century, however, the structure of British law was changed to reflect a less severe approach to those who stepped outside the boundaries of the family cell. Reflecting a change in the discourse of punishment from retribution to incarceration and reform, legal punishments for abortion and homosexuality were no longer punishable by death in Great Britain in 1867 and 1861, respectively. Arguably, the reason for this was not the inherent kindliness of the agents of the British state. As Foucault has suggested in *Discipline and Punish,* the most effective form of social control is that which forces subjects to perceive themselves as constantly under surveillance.[15] A number of discourses, again, worked in concert to effect this: the British state, with its newly created police force; neighbors and community, alert to those who might threaten their own well-being by stepping out of line and bringing attention to them; employers, watching workers to ensure efficient labor; the medical profession, joined with the nascent field of evolutionary science and criminal anthropology, observing "perverse" bodies and minds through the eyes of "science"; and God, mediated through religious discourse, the all-seeing eye/I who threatens to punish those who transgress the Law. The result was effective self-regulation, or internalization of the gaze.

In the case of the family cell in Ireland, it should not be assumed that the result of this self-regulation was a tendency to "follow the rules," however. Rather, the family cell regulated itself by keeping to itself; when social laws were transgressed in the family, self-preservation meant attempting to hide transgressions from the eyes of those who might punish them, whether it be the local community, the church, or the colonial authority.[16] The family cell thus remained the ideal unit group of society, while individual family cells regulated their public images and kept any instability under wraps. Backus provocatively argues that the "anxieties originating within the family are projected outside the family, perpetuating sectarian divisions" (6). Although this statement is made in reference to family within the gothic narrative, one could argue that this dynamic is necessary for preservation of any cell:

it is a method of concealing any instability within the cell in order to present the image of control. If the cell is stable, so too are the social institutions built upon it, and one can present to the world one's capacity to rule. Instabilities must therefore be constructed and treated as foreign—not only to the family, not only to one's political position, but also to the nation as a whole.

To accept this logic is to be contained by a discursive structure that excludes, silences, and injures a large portion of the population and strictly limits the public behaviors of all. But the family cell is a social structure that was firmly established and self-regulating; manipulation of that discourse was an effective means of control and reproduction, both literally and figuratively, of the social order. It is not surprising, then, that it remained as an idealized structure in both nineteenth- and twentieth-century Irish nationalist *and* unionist discourse and eventually was enshrined as the cornerstone of the new Irish nation-state.[17]

The Family Cell as Resistance: Mother Ireland and the Revolutionary Family Cell

Although the contraction of the family cell arose in part out of economic necessity, it found ideological support as a discourse of resistance. Even as early as the eighteenth century, two Irish responses to British colonial rule were Union—a political "marriage" between the British and the Irish—or union, marriage leading to the literal reproduction of the Irish people, particularly of Irish heroes or patriots. Both unionist/loyalist and Irish nationalist discourses presented the family as the bastion of moral righteousness and site of the reproduction of the cause, although Irish nationalist discourse, arguing simultaneously for tradition and emancipation, developed a more elaborate symbolic language of the family and particularly women's place within it.

Brian Merriman's famous Irish Gaelic poem *The Midnight Court*, praised by many modern readers for its relatively frank sexuality and its celebration of women's sexual power, is a manifesto for sexual reproduction through the family. The Catholic clergy, for instance, are admonished for their vows of celibacy:

> Má lagaigh an síolrach daonmhar, daona,
> I dtalamh dathaoibhinn fíorghlas Éireann,
> Is furas an tír d'athlíonadh de laocha
> D'uireaspa dlí gan bhrí, gan éifeacht.

> If the human race is really declining
> In the pleasant-hued, evergreen land of Ireland,
> It's easy to refill the land with heroes
> By a senseless pointless law repealing.[18]

The "jury" of the poem is encouraged to look to the children of Catholic clerics as evidence that they are already reproducing; implicitly, then, the text suggests that mere reproduction is not enough, that the reproduction of Irish heroes must take place through the legitimized family. Women in this poem have a "right" to sexual expression, but again this right is filtered through the family. The judge of the poem, a woman, lays down the statute at the end of the poem that "if a brow is unwrinkled, it is a crime / At thirty years to be without marital ties" (87, ll.1063–64).

Merriman's poem codes resistance to the economic deprivation being experienced by the Catholic Irish during the recurrent waves of famine in the late eighteenth century. The site of resistance to depopulation was the family cell, the place wherein Irish heroes could be reproduced. The family, in other words, became seen as a kind of revolutionary cell — but since it remained contained by the discourses that shaped it, its transgressive potential was and is limited. Nonetheless, the image of the revolutionary family cell was reinforced by Irish nationalist discourses that, like the British, saw Ireland as a woman who needed to be saved by her devoted sons from rape by the colonial invader. This discourse drew from the sovereignty goddess of early Irish myth who was able to confer kingship on a chosen leader and in the process transform from an old hag into a young woman.[19] The subtle shift in emphasis in nationalist versions of the myth, however, notably takes the agency away from the sovereignty goddess and puts it in the hands of the men of Ireland who must save a threatened woman-as-Ireland from mistreatment at the hands of the British invader. Such a construction idealizes a passive and pure female figure, the ideal woman of the house and keeper of the social order, and constructs the threat to both family and nation as external. The other side to this discourse, however, is that women are simultaneously constructed as a potential threat to the family unit. As in Yeats's famous nationalist play *Cathleen ni Houlihan,* her "trouble" is that she has "too many strangers in the house," and since she is written as a powerfully seductive force, there remains the implication that she promiscuously let them in herself.[20] She must be controlled; the marital trope of Britain as the colonial "husband" of the unruly Irish family echoes in the subtext of Irish nationalist discourse wherein the Irish man was expected to control both family cell and nation. The "unmanageable revolutionaries" of the Ladies Land League, the suffragists, even Inghinidhe na hÉireann and Cumann na mBan: all were threats to this idealized vision, and their presence in the public sphere was counteracted with celebrations of the mother of the rebel and a passive Mother Ireland, images that simultaneously idealized women's place in the private sphere and attempted to limit their public appearances to the merely inspirational and iconographic.[21]

The Public, the Private, and the Family Cell

This brief history of the family cell in Ireland brings me back to the terminology that has so often shaped legal and political discussions of gender, sexuality, and the family, in Ireland and elsewhere in the West: *public* and *private*. Since the rise of the discourse of civic humanism, the public sphere has been invoked and often celebrated as the place in which political debate and action happens; the private sphere has generally been described as the site of the individual and the family. As I suggest throughout this book, however, the separation between the two spheres is illusory, a fact that must be acknowledged if there is hope for a vital public sphere.

In the introduction to the collection of essays entitled *The Phantom Public Sphere*, Bruce Robbins explores the changing meanings of the terms "private" and "public" in philosophical-political tracts, starting with discussions in the 1920s and continuing to present-day struggles with the terms and the ideals they represent on both ends of the political spectrum. He encourages, instead of a wholesale rejection of the public/private dichotomy, a recognition of and attention to "the actual multiplicity of distinct and overlapping public discourses, public spheres, and scenes of evaluation that already exist, but that the usual idealizations have screened from view," ultimately hoping to tease out a notion of the public that "would be adequate to the connectedness of power."[22]

An admirable goal. But can a public sphere in which multiple discourses and bodies have agency, equal respect, and freedom without violence be imagined within the ways "private" and "public" are currently invoked? Robbins states summarily that "the lines between public and private are perpetually shifting, as are the tactical advantages of finding oneself on one side or another" (xv). Surveying the tensions between private and public outlined by feminist critics Catharine MacKinnon, Nancy Fraser, Rosalyn Deutsche, and Iris Marion Young—in short, how private and public are both terms invoked strategically to reify patriarchal relations — Robbins asserts that "feminist efforts would seem better aimed at the immediately disputable power to redraw the public/private line rather than the utopian goal of effacing all such lines" (xvi). Such a claim, however, does not address the similarities in MacKinnon's, Fraser's, Deutsche's, and Young's arguments and thus the underlying problems with the invocation of the public/private binary. All these theorists point to the ways in which the public/private dichotomy, because of the very slipperiness Robbins and others want to celebrate, relies on a not-so-slippery set of gendered power relations. For instance, Catharine MacKinnon, in *Toward a Feminist Theory of the State*, warns of the difficulties with using the language of "choice" to combat anti-abortion legislation. Although the goal of securing women's agency is admirable, the language of the U.S. *Roe v. Wade* decision links women's personal reproductive choices with privacy; so too does the Irish *McGee v. The Attorney General* decision, which links the right to choose contraception with marital privacy in particular and which draws explicitly on U.S. definitions of privacy. MacKinnon argues that "privacy is by no means a gender-neutral concept"; the liberal notion of protection of privacy assumes that, within the private sphere, all individuals are free and equal, which, as many women recognize, is not the case. As she argues, "for women the measure of the intimacy has been the measure of the oppression. This is why feminism has had to explode the private. This is why feminism has seen the personal as the political. . . . Feminism confronts the fact that women have no privacy to guarantee."[23] She suggests that we need to recognize the extent to which abortion issues have never been wholly "private" nor wholly "choices."

Taking the critique further, Nancy Fraser has effectively exposed the gender system underlying the often-invoked Habermasian model of public/private relations.[24] Jurgen Habermas distinguishes between not only public and private but also "lifeworld," the shared assumptions and values of a group, and "system." The nuclear family is a private lifeworld institution, and the (official) economy is a private system; the public sphere of debate and political participation is a public lifeworld institution, and the official administration of the state is a public system. Habermas criticizes the "colonization" of the private lifeworld by the systems of the official economy and the state, particularly in the late capitalist welfare state. But, as Fraser points out, the private lifeworld — the nuclear family — is by no means originally separate from and unaffected by these systems. Fraser complicates Habermas's model by suggesting the extent to which gender already informs not only the private life-world but also the participatory model of democracy celebrated by Habermas. As Fraser suggests, gender structures all of the systems and lifeworld institutions Habermas names. His model occludes our recognition of the ways these systems depend upon the patriarchal model of familial relations that defines the private lifeworld and its members' ability to participate in and affect the public sphere. The economy (a "private system") as well as the public sphere is thus exposed as already gendered. Habermas might argue that this gendering is a result of the colonization of lifeworld by system (the state in the form of public policy), but such an argument assumes that systems are not informed by lifeworlds. The language of public debate (a lifeworld sphere) is most certainly gendered, as feminist cultural critics have been pointing out for years; this is certainly no less true in Ireland than elsewhere. So-called private sexual relations serve as a foundation upon which the public sphere, both lifeworld and system, is built and reproduced. Patriarchal heterosexuality—which, as Judith Butler has argued, creates the gender system—is in itself a system that cuts across public and private lifeworlds and systems.[25]

In short, the family cell, as both lifeworld and system, shapes and controls agency within and between the private and public spheres. The family cell is a regulatory ideology, one that defines roles and choices. Those who step outside the ideal are pilloried in the public sphere or confined to silence in the private sphere; in this way, national discourses—whether of a loyalist Ulster, a revolutionary Ireland, or the Irish nation-state—contain internal challenges and reproduce themselves. Their main instrument in this process, I would argue, is *information*, a concept to which I turn next. Information can cut across public/private lines, sometimes in a liberatory way; but when the distinction between public and private is exploited, information operates as a system of oppression.

Information and the Cell

It is not coincidental that the family cell bears more than a passing resemblance to the revolutionary cell. In both cases, social, economic, and political pressures create a small, guarded group committed to self-preservation and self-reliance in the face of an oppressive political and economic structure. Repressive British laws, from the first statutes of

Kilkenny in the fourteenth century to the successive Emergency Acts in Northern Ireland in the twentieth century, meant that open networks of political association were out of the question for those interested in challenging the existing political structures in Ireland. Revolutionary cells, whether loyalist or republican, are guarded sites of resistance; each cell is kept deliberately small to reduce the chance that one individual or cell can bring down the larger network of cells when exposed.

The difference between the family cell and the revolutionary cell, however, is their relationship to the nation-state. The nation-state is invested in preserving the family "as the fundamental unit group of society," to quote, for instance, the Irish Constitution.[26] The family cell is concerned with self-preservation; self-preservation means opportunities for financial advancement and security for one's "own," not for the community as a whole. The tightened kinship bonds of the family cell, in short, promote the interests of capitalism by narrowing accessible routes to self-preservation and in turn promote the interests of a nation-state intent both on surviving and thriving within global capitalism and maintaining national sovereignty.

The revolutionary cell, on the other hand, ostensibly hopes to overthrow the current political system. In the case of Irish republicans from the nineteenth century onward, this has often meant a stated goal of a more equitable system of property and social relations. For both Irish republicans and Ulster unionists/loyalists, it means a reformulation of the nation-state. After the revolution, however, without a change in the limited nationalist vision of the family cell, the current system merely reproduces power relations: to reappropriate Yeats, as I like to do, "the beggars have changed places, but the lash goes on," and those in charge of the new nation-state find it necessary to police the private sphere in the name of national security.[27]

The circulation of information about the ideal nation and the nation-state, particularly that which threatens to expose internal vulnerabilities and abuses, must thus be controlled in order to ensure their reproduction. The agents of the nation and nation-state control information through their own kind of "informing." Information, or "knowledge communicated concerning some particular fact, subject, or event," works to inform, or "to give form to, put into form or shape . . . mould, or train" not only the family cell but also the individual subject within it.[28] A variety of discourses informs within the national and familial context, particularly religious discourse, which defines and shapes gender roles, and nationalist discourses, which refine the former and encourage appropriate behaviors for members, whether Irish or British, republican or loyalist.

Of course, to "inform" also means "to lay or exhibit information, bring a charge or complaint." To inform and to inform *against* are closely related: whether the agent is the state denying access to abortion information or an individual subject informing on another's political activities, "informing" helps to define the boundaries of the nation, the family cell, and the individual subject. The security of the nation thus depends on the control of information and informers.[29] Agents of the nation/state can use the threat of "information," or exposure of personal details, to secure their own self-interest. But nationalist discourses, whether in the hands of revolutionaries or the state, can only manipulate information by maintaining a strict division between public and private. Without those distinctions, informing loses its negative power, and subjects can move freely in the public sphere, offering alternatives to a nationalist discourse based on a limited and limiting notion of the family cell.

The family cell also has those who inform against it, the family member who exposes the so-called private family's workings to the attention of the public: the abused wife who informs on her husband, for instance, or the queer child who exposes his family's nonheteronormativity, or the pregnant daughter who names her own father as the father of her child. Nationalist discourse must attempt to contain the threat of these potential informers by constructing them as foreign bodies in the cell, pathological invaders threatening the very coherence of the cell. But informing, I suggest, is the only strategy for changing the status quo. The model of informing of which I speak hopefully here is not one that enforces and abuses the public/private distinction as it is currently structured; it is not one that merely reproduces ideologies of containment in order to reproduce bodies and labor for the existing social order. Rather, this kind of informing cuts across public/private lines to destabilize a limited vision of the family cell as the only appropriate private social model and in so doing offers more people both the benefits of the private sphere and access to the public. It is the kind of informing that invigorates the public sphere with new voices—and more information. Ailbhe Smyth, in her foreword to the queer-positive short story collection *Alternative Loves,* writes of the connection between literature and politics, her "strong sense that tangible social and political change is never achieved without the ability to imagine the world otherwise, to find the language which can give shape and substance to our unnameable, and thus unnamed, longings." Informing, I would suggest, provides the first step in offering the language to, in her words, "imagine the world otherwise."[30]

Although this project focuses on Irish politics, this book is aimed at an interdisciplinary audience—not only those working in Irish studies but also a larger audience interested in gender, sexuality, nationalism, the public and private spheres, and the relationship between these categories of analysis and action. By reading a broad variety of texts and in turn creating one myself, I hope to add to the positive process of informing I celebrate above. Texts are an accessible and essential part of the cultural, social, economic, and political fabric and are constitutive as well as representative of that fabric. Literary texts, for instance, can mediate between the discourse of intimacy and public discourse, challenging their boundaries and limitations. As Edna Longley has put it, imaginative literature "trellises the harsh girders with myriad details" (194), complicating large abstractions with intimate and local particularities that, even if not mimetic, are more honest for their specificity. But I do not believe that creative literature should be the only focus of textual analysis: political texts can offer insights into the shaping and deployment of discourse; and historiography and theory, including my own, can reveal patterns of events and representational strategies. All of these texts work together to produce the productive exchange of "informing." I also heed the warning of theorist Steven Seidman, however, who suggests that critiques that are not "institutionally situated" edge toward mere "textual idealism"—that is, they may shape future texts, but not real politics. By actively situating theoretical concerns in practice, I follow the lead of scholars such as Lauren Berlant, Gloria Anzaldua, Ailbhe Smyth, and others who have encouraged dialogue not only among scholars in different academic disciplines but between scholars and activists. In doing so, I hope to provide not only critique but a productive political intervention.

The first chapter, "Foreign Bodies: Representations of Homosexuality and the Irish Body Politic," builds on the theoretical and historical outline of this introduction by exploring the ways nationalist discourses treat homosexuality. The first part of the chapter examines Irish nationalist discourses that construct homosexuality as a specifically "foreign" threat, focusing in particular on responses to Roger Casement, an Anglo-Irishman charged with treason due to his part in the 1916 Easter Rising, who lost the support of Irish nationalists and was ultimately hanged when diaries were circulated that detailed his homosexual encounters. The chapter then traces the deployment of the construction of the homosexual-as-foreigner throughout the twentieth century, first in the debates over the decriminalization of homosexuality in Great Britain, Northern Ireland, and the Republic; then in representations of lesbians in Irish feminist writing; and finally in the controversy surrounding the Irish Lesbian and Gay Organization's request to march in the New York St. Patrick's Day parade. Using materials from these cultural moments, I investigate the particular political and cultural logic — a strategic logic based on the notion of the family cell — that requires nations to exclude homosexuality as an acknowledged possibility for their "true" subjects, even if it means excluding them from the body politic. I also analyze the responses to this homophobic discourse by writers in the North and South — including texts by Northern Irish and Irish novelists Stephen Birkett, June Levine, and Edna O'Brien and filmmaker Neil Jordan. Through close analysis of these narratives, I show how writers seemingly resistant to the nationalist silencing of feminist and homosexual narratives can reinforce the image of queer-as-foreigner, the hierarchizing of freedoms, and the privatization of the politics of sexuality that characterizes nationalist discourse.

Chapter 2, "Fetal Ireland: Reproduction, Agency, and Irish National Discourses," builds on the political implications of the discourse of foreignness examined in the first chapter and explores the rhetorical similarities between Irish nationalist discourse and anti-abortion discourse in the Republic and Northern Ireland through examinations of political debates, political pamphlets, short stories, novels, film, and historiography. I suggest that, just as the fetus is constructed as a pure potential citizen, threatened by women who attempt to exercise control over reproduction, the Republic of Ireland has been constructed as an autonomous but vulnerable fetus, threatened from without by Europe and, more generally, by feminist discourse. Any threat to the secure reproduction of the ideal citizen of the nation — any attempt to breach the family cell — means that the advocates of national reproduction must work, and have worked, to contain women's reproductive agency through regulation of the private sphere, as evidenced through the abortion amendments, the Kerry Babies Case in the 1980s, the X Case in 1992, legislation and activism following the X Case in the 1990s, and the recent return to these issues by the Irish government. These events suggest that women's reproductive concerns are central to the image of Ireland as moral haven, free from foreign meddling. The centrality of abortion to the Maastricht

Treaty debates in Ireland suggests that the impact of these discursive connections between Ireland and the fetus have affected not only women's agency but also Ireland's political and economic situation, as recent European Economic Community (EEC) debates reveal. The chapter ends with an analysis of the repercussions of these events and of strategies to contain women's agency in contemporary Northern Ireland politics, particularly on the short-lived debates in July 2000 about extending to Northern Ireland the abortion laws passed in Great Britain in 1967.

Chapter 3, "Stag/nation: Information, Space, and the Numbers Game of the North," places the book and its theoretical concerns within the ongoing debate about the political status of Northern Ireland. In particular, I argue that the exclusion of voices from the public sphere and from political agency threatens the success of the peace process and the formation of a new and effective government for Northern Ireland. The current process, according to the Good Friday Agreement, is founded on and reinforces the assumption that there are only two communities in Northern Ireland, unionist and nationalist, and the violence in Northern Ireland has tended to encourage onlookers and politicians to make this assumption. This outlook, however, only fuels cycles of violence in the North; it allows each of those communities to see itself as under threat from the other, reinforces the family cell as the only model of resistance, and ignores the violence exercised on a large part of its population in the name of internal policing. By making common cause across communities, queer and feminist discourses not only decentralize the familist model of nationalisms but potentially destabilize the two-community model that has for so long shaped Northern politics. But they can only do so, I suggest, if they refuse to accept private and public spheres shaped solely by the cell model, an exclusionary model of identity that merely reproduces hierarchy, containment, and inevitable conflict.

1

Foreign Bodies
Representations of Homosexuality and the Irish Body Politic

Not everything in the heterosexual garden is lovely.
—Baroness Gaitskell, House of Lords debate on
decriminalizing homosexuality, 1965

Sexuality, particularly homosexuality, has occupied an uncomfortable place in the country that has, however hesitantly, counted among its children Oscar Wilde, Roger Casement, Eva Gore-Booth, and Kate O'Brien. "Place" is a metaphor that I use consciously, for homosexuality has troubled the notions of nation and "Irishness," concepts that themselves are constructed with particular attention to space and place as well as history and narrative. Like gender, sexuality does not confine itself within familial or national borders. Any identity category potentially troubles the national border by threatening the primacy of national identity, but homosexuality in particular threatens the stability of the nation and state for at least two major reasons. First, the very instability and specific historical contingency of the concept of homosexuality makes the category more fluid than most and thus brings into question the coherence of all identity categories. Second, homosexuality does not fit neatly within the discourse of bourgeois nationalism, since it threatens the reproduction of the heterosexual family cell that serves as the foundation of the nation-state. This threat is perceived to be literal, insofar as homosexuals are seen not to reproduce; but just as important, homosexuals and homosexual unions challenge the inevitability and

security of the notion of the family cell as the only "natural" and fundamental unit group of society.[1] Consequently, the discourses of both Irish
and Ulster nationalisms, until very recently, have excluded homosexuality; when homosexuality does enter these discourses, it does so as a
sign of foreign corruption and disintegration. As Carl Stychin has put it
in his discussion of European national discourse, "same sex sexuality is
deployed as the alien other, linked to conspiracy, recruitment, opposition to the nation, and ultimately a threat to civilization" (9).

This chapter thus examines Irish and British nationalist narratives
that construct homosexuality as a "foreign" threat. I begin with an analysis of Kieran Rose's *Diverse Communities*, a history of gay activism in
the Republic of Ireland that introduces the notion of the queer-as-
foreigner as it emerged in Ireland at the end of the nineteenth century.[2]
This concept is manifested in representations of Roger Casement, an
Anglo-Irishman charged with treason due to his part in the 1916 Easter
Rising, who lost the support of Irish nationalists and was ultimately
hanged when diaries were circulated that detailed his homosexual encounters. Starting with representations of Casement, I study the discursive construction of the queer-as-foreigner during crisis periods in the
twentieth century, including representations of male homosexuals in
Britain during the early years of the Cold War, the Democratic Unionist's
"Save Ulster from Sodomy" campaign during the struggles for unionist
sovereignty in the late 1970s, the legal construction of male homosexuals in the court cases concerning decriminalization in the North and the
Republic, and various representations of the Irish Lesbian and Gay Organization (ILGO) in New York in the 1990s. What emerges, first in representations of male homosexuals and then in representations of queers
in general, is a picture of the homosexual as an agent who personifies the
breakdown first of the family cell and then of the borders of the nation-
state, particularly when those within the borders believe themselves to
be under siege. The concept of the homosexual as a foreign body in the
family cell, a free-floating moral contaminant, reveals a profound anxiety not only about sexual identity but also about the stability of the na-
tion/state and the security of its borders. In all of these cases, the nationalist discourse about homosexuality is aimed at containment of the
threat of national breakdown, and it does so by containing queer agency
and repressing queer voices.

Throughout the chapter, I also analyze queer, feminist, and queer-
positive responses to this homophobic discourse. At their most limiting,
these responses, intentionally or not, merely reproduce the privatization

of the politics of sexuality that characterizes nationalist discourse. At their most hopeful, however, these responses insist on a wider vision of the public sphere, one not shaped and contained by a fettered vision of the family cell.

Competing Traditions: Nationalism and Homosexuality

To begin, then, with an optimistic vision of the status of queers in Ireland: in the last twenty years, the legal acceptance of gays and lesbians has increased at an impressive rate. In the Republic, the final step in the decriminalization of male homosexuality in June 1993 was, according to gay activist Kieran Rose, "enthusiastically welcomed in both Houses of the Oireachtas." Rose notes further that "the Government . . . chose the more radical option, which, in the words of the leaked memo, 'would in effect equate, for the purposes of the law, homosexual and heterosexual behavior.'" This bill was the result of over twenty years of gay rights advocacy, advocacy that, in part, linked itself to the feminist movement for support and modeling.[3]

Rose's pamphlet argues that the radical changes in Irish official policy toward gays and lesbians are founded in "positive traditional Irish values arising from the anti-colonial struggle reinvigorated and amplified by the new social, cultural and economic influences of the 1960s onwards" (3). Rose invokes Irish traditionalism as the basis for social change, a surprising move, perhaps, given the frequency with which "traditional Irish values" have been the measure against which Irish conservative nationalists have held contemporary Irish culture and found it wanting. He explains: "The perception of the Irish people as irredemiably [*sic*] 'backward' on sexual and social issues was an idea that GLEN [Gay and Lesbian Equality Network] refused to accept. While there are obvious contradictions in Irish attitudes, GLEN knew that there was a tradition of tolerance, which was benign, and based on a belief in fairness and justice. GLEN knew that there were real and positive traditional Irish values, arising from the struggle against colonialism and for civil, religious and economic rights, which could be activated, and the demand for equality was attuned to this heritage" (4). By equating "traditional Irish values" and "heritage" with "tolerance," "justice," "fairness," and struggles for rights, GLEN linked the telos of liberation from oppression that nationalists share with other Irish activists, such as feminists and socialists. This rhetorical strategy was an attempt to refigure a simplistic concept of Irish "tradition" often evoked by conservative nationalists, a tradition perhaps best characterized by Eamon DeValera's (in)famous 1943 St. Patrick's Day speech in which he conjures visions of his ideal Ireland full of "cozy homesteads," "athletic youths," "sturdy children," and "comely maidens." At the same time, GLEN hoped to harness the appeal of words like "tradition" and "heritage" that were and are so often linked to that vision.

In order to pursue this rhetorical strategy, Rose notes but smoothes over references to Irish nationalist homophobia, returning consistently to the claim that nationalist homophobia is a legacy of British colonialism. This claim is a compelling one, potentially echoing Ashis Nandy's claims that nationalist movements often respond to colonialism within the discursive limits set by the colonizer. Rose states that "the late-nineteenth century also saw a deepening hostility towards male homosexuality from what Lynne Segal (1990) has described as 'the late-Victorian storm-troopers of a new aggressive masculinity'" (6). He then cites Jeffrey Weeks's explanation of the homosexual purges of the 1880s and the 1885 legislation criminalizing sexual practices between men as part of the general British concern with "imperialism and national decline" (6). This brief history suggests that homophobia was an important part of the British attempt to maintain its own national self-image. But he also goes on to mention a disturbing period in Ireland's own nationalist history: "The Irish nationalist press pursued 'homosexual scandals' from the opposite direction, as a means of undermining certain highly-placed officials in the colonial administration in Dublin, one of whom was said to bear 'the odium of contaminating the running stream of Irish moral purity by stirring up the stink of pollution planted by foreign hands' (Breen 1990). It is significant that Irish nationalist ideology developed during such a homophobic period in European history."[4] It is indeed significant; Rose's juxtaposition of the similar English and Irish responses to male homosexuality suggest that both have at least occasionally shared a repressive and patriarchal ethos.

Irish nationalist homophobia is perhaps not difficult to explain, however, even if it is difficult to justify. Ashis Nandy has famously suggested that the discourse of European colonialism, by describing the colonized as feminine (and thus disorderly, weak, and in need of masculine rule), encourages a response of "hypermasculinity" on the part of the colonized, a kind of masculinity or "manliness," as Adrian Frazier has described it, defined by "excellence in the propagation of new citizens, in combat against aliens, in the expansion of an industrial economy, and in the regulation of respectability in the home."[5] Other forms of masculinity, Frazier suggests, were available, particularly in the sphere of cultural nationalism; but nationalism, as "a quasi-military movement, . . . had to create unity by crushing forms of diversity within its borders and by entering into rivalries for spheres of power beyond those borders" (10). Other ways of imagining masculinity were available, but their public circulation was circumscribed by nationalist interests as a form of self-protection. Oscar Wilde provides a case in point: near the end of the nineteenth century, as Alan Sinfield has argued, effeminacy and male homosexuality were linked in the course of the Wilde trials — and Wilde, for all of his cosmopolitanism, was Irish.[6] The Irish nationalist desire to gain distance from male homosexuality is not surprising, then, given the extent to which homosexuality could be used as further evidence of Irish "disorder" and depravity, a discursive construction that the British invoked to justify their rule and against which the nationalists had been fighting for years. Following this logic, the Irish nationalist press's pursuit of homosexual scandals among colonial officials could be seen as an attempt to hold the British to their own standard of "morality."

What is more interesting is that both the British colonial powers and the Irish nationalists wrote homosexuality as a kind of foreign "pollution." This characterization would be repeated in the early years of the AIDS crisis, when the general populace denied the presence of AIDS in Ireland, and, concurrently, right-wing Christian groups such as Family Solidarity castigated homosexuals as carriers.[7] Such a conflation of "sin" and disease, and thus contagion, can be traced at least as far back as the medieval period.[8] The term "buggery" itself derives from "Bulgarian," a name given to a sect of eleventh-century heretics (OED); this etymology suggests the longstanding desire to project male homosexuality elsewhere, to locate it in another geographical place. Homosexuality's supposed foreignness and contagiousness, then, combine to suggest a threat to the heterosexual family cell that serves as a foundation for the nation. Implicit in that threat, however, are two assumptions: that homosexuality is never "native"; and that the heterosexual family cell, and by extension the nation, are susceptible to "infection." The concept of the homosexual as a foreign body, an infectious agent in the family cell, thus reveals a profound anxiety not only about sexual identity but also about the stability of the nation and state and the security of their borders.

This anxiety was in evidence, as Rose's history attests, when Irish nationalists were working to found the new Irish state. As Irish nationalists struggled to achieve political self-determination, what constituted that "self" was still being debated. The ideal geopolitical boundaries of the state were fixed but had not been established, and the Irish nation, like any nation, was composed of a complex and sometimes conflicting set of ideologies, histories, and allegiances. At this originary point, prior to statehood, "Ireland" and "Irishness" as concepts were both contested and particularly vulnerable to perceived attack. And a particular example of the volatile nature of the "scandal" of homosexuality in such a context is the case of Roger Casement.

Perverted Justice: Roger Casement and the Treason of Ambiguity

Sir Roger Casement, diplomat and humanitarian, is best known in Irish history for his attempt to supply the Irish nationalist forces with arms from Germany for the Easter Rising in 1916. The boat carrying the arms was intercepted and scuttled; Casement landed in Kerry to call off the rising but was captured before the message could be sent. He was then taken to London and tried on charges of treason. His lawyer, Serjeant Sullivan—the last Queen's Serjeant in Ireland—was a conservative and a unionist, which ensured a less-than-friendly relationship between him and Casement. His ineffective defense was mounted based on a point of grammar in a fourteenth-century statute; its success rested on whether or not there was a comma in that document.

With Casement's defense already compromised by such an odd and precarious legal strategy, he was then attacked by the press when his diaries, detailing his homosexual encounters, were discovered and circulated among politicians and potential supporters of his reprieve both in Great Britain and the United States. When Sullivan questioned him about the diaries, it is claimed that Casement admitted and defended his homosexuality.[9] Ultimately, Casement's defense did not succeed, and he was hanged for treason in August of 1916.[10]

Casement's actions—collaboration with the enemy in a time of war—certainly would have been enough to justify the accusations of treason. But his own defense lawyer suggests a further justification: treason and homosexuality were intimately connected. He asserted that "Casement was not completely normal and one of the abnormalities of his type is addiction to lamentable practices. He had the further affliction of the craving to record erotica and this horrible document was in the hands of the crown."[11] What is included under the rubric of "lamentable practices" in this instance is not wholly clear, but the structure of the

sentence suggests that it could include the tendency toward Irish nationalism as likely as the tendency toward homosexual acts. That is, if
the "lamentable practices" were homosexual acts only, the normal rhetorical construction would be that Casement had the "further affliction
of the craving to record *them*"; that Sullivan specifies the diaries as a
"further affliction" suggests that the "lamentable practices" encompass
the whole lot. Casement's "type," then, is the "abnormal" Irish rebel/
homosexual. Casement's acceptance of physical-force nationalism and
his secret collaboration with the Germans on behalf of the Irish corre-
spond, in the eyes of the British, with his secret homosexual life. And
their decision to circulate the diaries — to give them "private publicity,"
as critic Lucy McDiarmid has put it — set the terms for the Irish nationalist response.[12]

Were the "Black Diaries" forged?[13] This is certainly a fascinating
question, and several book-length works have been devoted to it, both
before and after the diaries were available for public study.[14] With the
1997 publication of the Black Diaries, the critical debate about authenticity was given new fuel. But the answer to the question of authenticity
is not one of the concerns of this chapter; regardless of the authenticity
of the diaries, the debates around the issue of authenticity suggest the
extent to which Casement, as Kieran Kennedy has put it, "became a
spectacular embodiment of post-Edwardian England's and Ireland's
anxieties about masculinity and male sexuality" — and, I would add, national identity.[15]

The response of Casement's friends and supporters to the diaries was
general disbelief and active campaigning to "clear his name," both of the
charges of treason and of the "accusations" of homosexuality. But, despite urging from friends, Casement would not lie and claim that he had
been on his way to stop the Easter Rising rather than participate in it; nor
is it wholly clear whether he denounced the diaries. Nonetheless, many
of his supporters persistently clung to the claim of forgery. For Irish nationalists to accept that Casement was an "Irish patriot" — and, particularly, to claim him as a martyr — required that his homosexuality be
pushed back into the closet or denied.[16] Both the British and the Irish
made his sexuality foreign, either by denying it and accepting his patri-
otism (the Irish nationalist response) or by accepting both his Irish nationalism and his sexuality as evidence of the same treasonous problem.

William Butler Yeats, among others, enthusiastically accepted the
claim that the diaries were forged. In a letter to Ethel Mannin written in
November of 1936, Yeats writes, "I am in a rage. I have just got a book

published by the Talbot Press called *The Forged Casement Diaries*. It is by a Dr. Maloney I knew in New York and he has spent years collecting evidence. He has proved that the diaries, supposed to prove Casement 'a Degenerate' and successfully used to prevent an agitation for his reprieve, were forged. Casement was not a very able man but he was gallant and unselfish, and had surely his right to leave what he would have considered an unsullied name. I long to break my rule against politics and call these men criminals but I must not. Perhaps a verse may come to me, now or a year hence."[17] This is the first mention of Casement in Yeats's writing. It is worth noting what Yeats points out here: that the diaries prevented agitation for a reprieve. Though this is not strictly true — Casement's close friends kept up the fight until days before his death — it is true that the diaries prevented a more general outcry against his execution, despite their ostensible lack of relevance to the case at hand. But I will return to the issue of the diaries' relevance to Casement's treason. First, it is worth looking at the verses *The Forged Casement Diaries* inspired Yeats to write.

Yeats wrote two poems for Casement: "Roger Casement" and "The Ghost of Roger Casement," arranged respectively in *Last Poems*.[18] *Last Poems* gives a strong sense of Yeats's growing disillusionment with politics, both British and Irish, and both Casement poems show Yeats's anger at the British government's abuse of power. The first poem is addressed toward those who used the diaries to "blacken his good name": the "perjurer," "forger," "Spring Rice" (Sir Cecil Arthur Spring-Rice, British ambassador to America), and "all the troop / That cried it far and wide."[19] The poem, written for publication in one of the major Irish newspapers, is an appeal to the British to "make amends." A letter to Dorothy Wellesley suggests Yeats's tendency to combine the crime of treason with the evidence of homosexuality: "But the Casement evidence was not true as we know — it was one of a number of acts of forgery committed at that time. I can only repeat words spoken to me by the old head of the Fenians years ago. 'There are things a man must not do even to save a nation'" (*Letters*, 870). Presumably, the "nation" of which Yeats speaks is Great Britain, and the "things" are forgery and perjury: in this reading, Yeats accuses the British of trying to save their nation with "evidence" of Casement's homosexuality, even though the diaries were not "evidence" in any legal sense. But if the "nation" to which Yeats refers is Ireland, the statement presents an odd conflation of the sexual and political acts of which Casement was accused, a reading supported by the fact that the "nation" to which the Fenian (presumably John O'Leary) refers is Ireland. In either interpretation, Yeats conflates the two "guilts"—not at all surprising, given the extent to which the "crimes" of homosexuality and treason themselves were linked both rhetorically in Maloney's book and actually in the circumstances surrounding Casement's trial. That Wellesley, to whom he wrote the letter, was herself a lesbian seems not to have caused Yeats to censor his opinions; perhaps he even believed her, a protégé, to be a particularly apt audience for a warning about the dangers of combining sex and politics.

Adrian Frazier suggests that "Yeats sometimes envied homosexuals like Verlaine, while still conceiving them to be defective or immoral. . . . Creation was set against procreation, art against nature, and perversity against normality. . . . To be an artist, it was perhaps necessary to explore other ways of being male" (14). Frazier's provocative account of the alternative masculinities of major figures of the Irish literary renaissance might suggest that Yeats would have celebrated Casement's "perversity." But Frazier also describes a shift in Yeats from early representations of self and masculinity to "the middle Yeats, praiser of Don Juan and his sweaty thigh" who "achieves that missing sexual confidence and shuns his youthful effeminacy" (29). This is not to suggest that Yeats moved into homophobia as he aged, but rather that his ambivalence about private sexualities appears to have remained. Yeats's focus on Casement thus seems to have been on the latter's public life, although his writings about Casement show his discomfort with the relationship between Casement's private and public personae, between "perversity" and politics.

His discomfort apparently did not extend to Charles Stewart Parnell, whom he is presumably including in the "number of acts of forgery" to which he refers in his letter to Wellesley. Yeats supported Parnell, whose political life involved forgeries and evidence of sexual "misconduct."[20] Yeats's anger over the treatment of Parnell was directed both at the British government over the forgeries manufactured to knock him from political power via the Invincibles case and at the Irish clergy and other members of the Irish Parliamentary Party for agitating for Parnell to step down from his leadership position after he was named as co-respondent in the O'Shea divorce case. Yeats's reference in the letter to the Casement "forgeries" as political "evidence" against him gestures back to Parnell but in so doing suggests a blurring of the lines between two separate

legal cases against Parnell that involved accusations of sexual and political "sins." Yeats's recent reading of Henry Harrison's *Parnell Vindicated*, which helped inspire his Parnell ballad, would have further supported his tendency to see the two cases as similar. The Parnell letters
forged by Pigott, however, were evidence against him in the legal case
linking him to the Invincibles murders. The proof of forgery in that legal
case meant Parnell's reprieve; in the adultery case in which Parnell was
named co-respondent, however, there were no such forgeries to exoner-
ate him of accusations of sexual misconduct. Nonetheless, Yeats seems
to suggest in his letter to Wellesley that the Casement case is a repetition
of the same problem: a patriot brought down by British conspiracy, forgery, and popular opinion.[21]

   Although Yeats's view of the British is similar in both cases, his representation of the ostensible sexual misconduct in both is not. The poem
inspired by Parnell's case, "Come Gather Round Me Parnellites," cele-
brates Parnell's affair. The similarity in syntactic construction of the last
two lines of that ballad, "And Parnell loved his country / And Parnell
loved his lass" (*Poems*, 586, ll. 31–32), suggests a parallel, even a connection, between the two forms of loving. The literal and symbolic registers
are collapsed, as the loving of a woman becomes an understandably
masculine, virile corollary of loving a nation (as in loving Mother Ireland or Cathleen ni Houlihan). That Parnell actually loved an *English*
woman is, of course, not part of the poetic formula. In the Casement
poems, however, Yeats does not suggest that love for a man is coequal
with love of country; rather, the accusation of the former seems to pre-
clude the latter. The poems instead focus on accusation and anger at the
British government. It is, perhaps, significant that all three poems are
written in ballad form, but the last of them — "The Ghost of Roger Casement"—is the least "singable." Though it follows traditional ballad meter the most closely, the repetition of the refrain—"*The ghost of Roger
Casement / Is beating on the door*"—disturbs the rhyme scheme every time
it appears after the first stanza. The ghost meant to haunt the British also
haunts the poem; the meter and refrain, which on first glance make the
poem similar to a popular ballad, do not work together. Ironically, the
repetition of the refrain prevents the poem from being repeated as a
ballad.

   The poem serves, perhaps, as a metaphor for Casement himself: not
easily resolvable, awkward, not easily fit into prescribed categories; perhaps even a figure of fragmentation and disintegration. Casement's
biographers, especially those who wrote about him after the "Black

Diaries" were available for study, seem to agree upon such a character-ization.[22] B. L. Reid's biography *The Lives of Roger Casement* is perhaps the most interesting both in its representation of Casement's compli-cated personal and political identity and in its own ambivalence toward its subject. Even Reid's title suggests a fragmentation of narratives and selves; in his preface, he writes that "[Casement] was fragmented, and he was elusive: he was defined not by coherency but by complex ten-sions barely contained" (xv). Reid himself treats Casement's sexuality with an odd mixture of tolerance, clinical distance, judgmental criticism, and personal sympathy. In the appendixes in which he treats the issue of authenticity, for example, Reid refers to the question of Casement's sexual orientation as one that concerns his "purity," suggesting that ho-mosexuality is, by extension, "impure"; he also refers to the evidence of Casement's homosexuality as "negative" evidence (466, 468). He goes on, however, to write acceptingly that "I find nothing innately filthy-minded in any of this" (481). Again, seemingly derogating Casement's homosexuality, Reid quotes Ernley Blackwell's memorandum to the cabinet, which states that Casement "seems to have completed the full cycle of sexual degeneracy and from a pervert has become an invert — a woman, or pathic, who derives his satisfaction from attracting men and inducing them to use him."[23] He then responds in agreement that "Blackwell's statement is clinically if cruelly accurate," goes on to detail Casement's sexual habits, and notes that "more often than not he func-tioned primarily as the receiving or female partner" (465). While agree-ing with Blackwell's diagnosis, however, Reid takes issue with its tone, "its purse-lipped supercilious condemnatory delivery" that he argues "comes from the same Victorian habit of mind, puritanical, self-righteous, and wholly unimaginative, that leads a presumably more enlightened man of the generation of René MacColl still to call Casement a 'degen-erate,' a 'clandestine pervert,' a 'self-confessed pervert'" (465).

In a tone of acceptance, Reid continues: "Casement was not a pervert: he was an invert; and he was not a degenerate: he was a homosexual. He was a citizen of an alternative sexual world" (465). The language of citi-zenship in this context is striking and strange; one does not usually speak of "citizenship" in "sexual worlds." Reid's statement could be read generously as a sympathetic description of a radical position out-side of national familism. But it is also an implicit denial that Casement had either allegiance to, nor rights in, any other "world" beyond that of homosexuality. Casement does not, Reid implies, fit into the "normal" world comprised of national allegiances, identities, and politics.

The end of Reid's last chapter represents the extent to which Casement's citizenship in the "alternative world" of homosexuality frustrated any attempts to categorize him: "Casement's nature was divided to a depth just short of real pathology, of disastrous incoherence. Was he an Irishman or an Englishman; an Irish patriot or an English public servant; a countryman or a cityman; a man of the people or a gentleman; an Irish peasant or an Irish senator; an intellectual or an artist; an intellectual or a man of action; an idealist or a pragmatist; a sensualist or an anchorite; an African or a European; a Protestant or a Catholic; a man or a woman; a man or a boy? He did not know: he was all of them."[24] As this extensive list suggests, Casement—his "citizenship," nationality, class, sexuality, "gender"—did not fit neatly into the usual binaries; Reid does not even attempt to line up the terms in the list to suggest parallels between often-linked categories (Irishness, art, femininity, and sensuality, for instance). Reid does employ a pathologizing discourse when describing Casement, but the "disastrous incoherence" he describes is more than just that of homosexuality. As he moves toward a conclusion, Reid makes a particularly insightful observation: "his dividedness represented a whole culture, a whole era; strange as he was, he represented us all" (454). Reid, nearing the conclusion of the last chapter of Casement's life, seems to recognize that the fluidity and "incoherence" of Casement's identity is the fluidity and incoherence of *identity*. Though Reid goes on in his final lines to invoke Hamlet, "greatness," and "tragedy," this last insight is perhaps the most significant: he realizes, however briefly, that Casement embodies the tensions necessarily produced by exclusive identity categories and allegiances—tensions that may be especially visible in him, but that are also present in "us all."

Reid is one of the few who have had this epiphany, however, and to accept its implications fully can be a profoundly unsettling step. It is much easier to scapegoat those who seem to represent contradictions than to acknowledge that all identity categories and allegiances are inherently unstable, for to do the latter is to accept that the social, economic, and political structures built upon those categories—in this case, the nation and state—are also inherently unstable. Those who make this instability visible are thus liable to be described as unusual and as outsiders, allowing the nation and nation-state to maintain the illusion of stability and fixity. Casement was one of these people, and for this reason he was anathema to national security: for Great Britain, he was a literal security threat during wartime, but in the case of Ireland, he was and is still for some a threat to the secure reproduction of a coherent national self-image. The latter was particularly true in the period after 1916 during which Ireland was trying to establish itself as a sovereign, distinct, and independent power. Casement was and is a wild card; the threat he poses is that of the spy or informer, occupying a space simultaneously inside and outside the nation, the family cell, and even the revolutionary cell, a foreigner/native who in his mixed allegiances threatens to expose and destabilize everyone and everything and who therefore must be contained. Such assumptions lie at the heart of many discussions of homosexuality in a national context. With this in mind, it is perhaps not surprising that Sir Basil Thomson, in 1922, would entitle the book in which he discusses Casement *Queer People*. As Roger Sawyer notes, the "queer people" to which he refers are "forgers, traitors and spies" (1984, 8); but even by this time, "queer" had already begun to mean not only "strange" but also "homosexual." The links between sexuality and national treason had already been established.

"The Moral Bottom of Society": Decriminalization in Great Britain

The "alternative sexual world" that B. L. Reid describes Casement as inhabiting increasingly captured the attention of the British public even as the Casement "scandal" faded from the immediate attention of the Irish public. To understand the context both for the reception of Casement's diaries and the later Irish movements for homosexual law reform, it is worth taking what might seem like a detour into British politics and British homosexual law reform during a particularly volatile period in terms of the public discourse about male homosexuality. The connection between criminality and male homosexuality was to be examined most closely during the height of the Cold War, when the British government turned its attention to the question of whether homosexual acts should be decriminalized.[25] The political debates that ensued showed a desire to maintain the family cell and a desire to control the circulation of information that maintained both that cell and the nation/state. Both the logic of criminalization and the logic of law reform in Great Britain, I would argue, directly influenced the discourse about homosexuality in Ireland, North and South.

As Jeffrey Weeks suggests, law reform in Great Britain was facilitated by a variety of social factors, including the "ambiguous duality in the moral attitudes of the 1950s" that celebrated the "joyous merits of a secure family life" on one hand and emphasized, if in a somewhat veiled fashion, sexual pleasure and allure on the other.[26] But there were, as he also suggests, less abstract reasons for the reexamination of the laws. The late 1940s and early 1950s saw a great increase in the number of cases of indictable homosexual offenses, an increase that followed the appointment of a conservative director of public prosecutions, supported both by the Labour home secretary and the Tory home secretary. Examining these cases, government officials noted wildly disparate rates of prosecution as well as different degrees of severity in the punishment of homosexual offenses.

The increase in prosecutions was not the only reason male homosexuality had captured the attention of the government — and the public. In 1951 Guy Burgess and Donald Maclean, two Cambridge schoolmates who were in the employ of the Foreign Office and who had recently been discovered by British security forces to have been Soviet spies, mysteriously fled the country — a move, Rebecca West theorizes, deliberately planned by the Soviets to shake American confidence in British security organizations.[27] If West's theory is correct, the move was certainly a wise one. Neither man was likely to inspire confidence in American governmental circles: when sent by the Foreign Office to Washington, Burgess made a name for himself with his excessive drinking and was arrested three times; Maclean was, "even by American standards, a heavy drinker" (West, 220) and was known for getting involved in drunken brawls and other wild misbehavior. To add to this, in 1950 the United States government, particularly the State Department, had begun to purge itself of homosexuals in its ranks. According to the congressional document *Employment of Homosexuals and Other Sex Perverts in Government*, homosexuals were seen to be security risks because of their "emotional instability" and "the weakness of their moral fibre" (Weeks, 160). And Burgess and Maclean were homosexuals. Maclean was married but was known by many in governmental circles to have engaged in homosexual affairs, and Burgess was, by all accounts, hardly shy about his homosexuality.

The Burgess-Maclean affair raised public interest in homosexuality and confirmed the popular notion of homosexual men as decadent and untrustworthy. As Weeks has argued, male homosexuality was seen from the 1890s on as an indicator of the possible decline of the British Empire, a concept modeled in part on the belief that the Roman Empire fell because of the sins of lust and excess typified, in the popular view, by homosexuals (16–22). That Burgess and Maclean were graduates of Cambridge only added to the common conception of male homosexuality as an upper-class phenomenon, a notion popularized by the Wilde trials and reinforced as scandals involving highly placed public figures were exploited by the press. Throw into the political mix the fact that some pro-gay figures, such as Edward Carpenter and George Cecil Ives, were also outspoken idealistic socialists, and, more obviously, that Burgess and Maclean had made common cause with the foreign Communist enemy, and homosexuality seemed to many like a particularly dangerous threat to the stability of the nation.

Public attention was also turned to the situation of homosexual men with the press coverage of several trials in the early 1950s.[28] As Weeks describes in "Prelude to Reform," Lord Montagu, along with Kenneth Hume, a film director, was charged but not convicted of "indecently assaulting" two Boy Scouts in 1954. Montagu was to be retried. Peter Wildeblood, diplomatic correspondent for the *Daily Mail*, and Michael Pitt-Rivers, Lord Montagu's cousin, were arrested several weeks later on charges of indecency and also with conspiracy with Montagu to commit the crimes. The latter conspiracy charges, as Weeks suggests, were clearly an attempt to jeopardize Montagu's retrial. As he says, "at the trial of all three in April 1954, the prosecution offered an amazing display of prejudice and malice — and a careful loading of the dice" (161). He continues, "what emerged in this, as in other trials of the period, was the attempt to sustain the stereotype of male homosexuals as decadent, corrupt, effete and effeminate. And in this endeavor the state was aided by the popular press" (162).

But the Wildeblood-Montagu trial, as Stephen Jeffery-Poulter writes, exposed police abuses in the conviction of the men, such as illegal search and seizure, tampering with evidence, and the denial of access to legal counsel. It also became clear that the men who were "solicited" by Montagu, Wildeblood, and Pitt-Rivers were promised immunity in exchange for turning queen's evidence.[29] Public opinion was, therefore, split as a result of the affair. Many still believed that homosexuals were decadent and effete, but many — including some of the former — also believed that the state was not playing fair. As Weeks suggests, this trial in particular served as a "catalyst which revealed the inherent problems in the situation of homosexuals. Either the law had to be tightened up further, more rigorously and evenly applied . . . or it had to be reformed" (164).

The Home Office, anxious to calm the controversy, promised to put together a committee to examine the homosexual criminal code. But the promise did little to placate members of Parliament. The public attention to the Wildeblood-Montagu case spurred the first debates in Parliament on the issue of homosexuality and the law. Members' speeches echoed the division in public opinion: some believed the laws should be changed, either because they were ineffective in stopping male homosexuality or because government should not interfere in issues of private morality, whereas others believed that changes in the law would lead to more widespread male homosexuality and, ultimately, to the moral decline of Great Britain. In the words of the bishop of Southall, "Once a people lets its ultimate convictions go, then there can be no stopping half way, and the whole moral bottom is in danger of falling out of a society" (Jeffery-Poulter, 21).

The Home Office followed through with its promise and put together a committee in 1954, a few months after the Parliamentary debates. The Wolfenden Committee was varied in its makeup and in the opinions of its members and took a fairly level-headed approach to the issues that it was charged to address. The committee reported in September of 1957 and recommended (with some members offering their detailed reservations about certain recommendations) several changes in the law, including "that homosexual behaviour between consenting adults in private be no longer a criminal offense" ("the age of 'adulthood'" being "fixed at twenty-one") and "that buggery be re-classified as a misdemeanor" (as opposed to a felony).[30] As Weeks notes, "limited and conservative as the proposals were, they caused a whirlwind of controversy" (166), and the recommendations were shelved for several years until the political lobbying of the Homosexual Law Reform Society helped to bring attention back to the issue.

A first attempt to enact some of the recommendations of the Wolfenden report occurred in 1962, when Leo Abse brought a bill before Commons. That bill went nowhere, however, and it was not until 1965 that the issue was raised in Parliament again—this time by the Earl of Arran, Arthur Gore, in the House of Lords. The debates that ensued over the next two years offer some insight not only into the attitudes toward and history of homosexual law reform in Great Britain and eventually Northern Ireland, but also more broadly into the anxieties about identity, individual and national, that accompany the political treatment of homosexuality.

Much of the debate focused on whether homosexuality should be a crime as well as a sin; the latter was generally taken for granted both by pro- and anti-reform speakers. Both sides also tended to present heterosexuality as inextricably linked with love, family, and happiness, leaving homosexuality thus as a confusing, troubling "condition." Several of the speakers for the law reform asserted that homosexuality had been demonstrated by experts to be an uncontrollable condition, citing in particular the evidence in the Wolfenden report. The Earl of Arran asked, "will any man or woman in your Lordships' House tell us seriously that a man, out of perverseness — and I mean perverseness, not perversion — purposely renounces the joys of love with the opposite sex, the joys of having a wife, the joys of having children? . . . And is it even remotely possible that there could be half a million such obstinate men in Britain alone?"[31] G. R. Strauss echoed this sentiment in a 1966 speech to the Commons: "Homosexuals do not voluntarily give up the warmth and happiness of marriage, the conjugal home and the joy of children. It is not through choice that they are homosexuals" (Commons, 1966, 806). In short, that one could and would choose homosexuality over the heterosexual family was presented as unthinkable by a vast majority of those in favor of reform; the family cell was so firmly idealized that an appeal to its joys was treated as evidence.

As Roy Jenkins, who introduced the bill into Commons, argued, "in general [homosexuality] is, I am convinced, an involuntary deviation. . . . It is not a disease in the sense of being, in the majority of cases, subject to medical treatment. It is more in the nature of a disability than a disease and, of course, it is a grave disability for the individual" (Commons, 1966, 850)—a comment later quoted in 1977 by the Standing Commission on Human Rights in Northern Ireland as a reason for changing the law there to conform with that of the rest of Great Britain.[32] Jenkins continued, "It leads to a great deal of loneliness and unhappiness and to a heavy weight of guilt and shame. It greatly reduces the chance of the individual finding a stable and lasting emotional relationship." "Stability" is a key word here, I would argue; as in the Casement case, the essential "instability" of the homosexual was a grave fear. Even though Jenkins was wholly in support of the law, his choice of words was echoed by several of those who spoke against law reform — most notably, perhaps, William Shepherd:

> The House, while being careful to look at this issue with compassion and even with liberality, ought . . . to be careful to ensure that it is not misled by propaganda of a wildly distorted kind. Neither must the House be unmindful of the nature of homosexuals themselves.
>
> I do not want the House to accept what I say. I simply want the House to accept what was said by Richard Hauser, who was

appointed by the Home Secretary to conduct an investigation into homosexuality. Richard Hauser has done a lot to help homosexuals and he says that he knows no minority — he is one of a minority himself; he is a Jew — among whom self-pity and self-righteousness are so rampant. He knows no minority which is so lacking a sense of values outside its own circle, no minority which is so bereft of loyalty to its country. In looking at this issue, we have to bear in mind the essential nature of homosexuality and of homosexuals. (Commons, 1966, 810)

Shepherd suggests that homosexuals do have choice, and that they choose not to enter into heterosexual relationships because they "are people who are seeking sexual gratification without responsibility" (815). The homosexual, in short, is unstable because he *does* have choice, choice that he exercises without loyalty to the family cell and thus to the nation. As Hauser, to whom Shepherd appeals, wrote, "having no wives or children to tie them, they can travel easily, and wherever they go they can be sure of making 'interesting' contacts"; "'interesting' contacts" in the context of Hauser's description of the homosexual "underworld" could suggest not only sexual contacts but also other "unorthodox people who [laugh] behind society's back" — that is, others who might be disloyal to the nation in thought or action.[33]

Homosexuals, then, are mobile, not confined by the family physically or "morally," and by extension not confined by the nation, either. They are not easily contained. This concern about the uncontainability of male homosexuality finds outlet in discussions about homosexual proselytizing. Interestingly, in the one of the very few mentions of lesbians in the Parliamentary debates, Shepherd asserted that "lesbians do no physical damage by their acts. They are not proselytisers as homosexuals are and, on the whole, they find it agreeable to live together for long periods of time" (816). That is, although lesbians do not compose a heterosexual family cell, they do not threaten the institution through proselytizing. In short, they contain themselves.

Proselytizing emerges often in both the Commons and Lords debates, and the way the issue was treated shows that the discussions about the uncontainability of homosexuality barely mask the fearful recognition that heterosexual identity is itself unstable. As the question about the appropriate age of consent arose, many expressed their concerns that, as W. R. Rees-Davies so wonderfully put it, "those who really understand this subject . . . know that there is no cure for the bugger who has been buggered from sixteen onwards" (Commons, 1967, 1423). Fears about proselytizing, of course, imply that proselytizing is effective, that one can be convinced to forego the heterosexual path. This belief was in part based on the Kinsey reports, released in 1948, that introduced to a wide audience the spectrum theory of sexuality and introduced the possibility that one's sexuality might not be immutable. Reid's comments about Casement resonate loudly here; implicit is the recognition that sexual identity is not containable through legislation.

The discussion of the effectiveness of proselytizing, however, was wholly externalized and separated from *individual* members' experience — even though the debates echoed with untold stories about homosexual experiences during school days or on the front, occasionally alluded to in the typical "I know of a man . . ." style, and "accusations" of other members' personal homosexual knowledge occasionally flew. In this situation, an individual's knowledge was used as a weapon against him; if one spoke with knowledge about homosexuality, one was "one of them" and therefore discredited. Authority came from speaking not with inside knowledge, for to admit to homosexuality, even to admit to a one-time homosexual encounter, was to cross the line between the private and the public and to deauthorize oneself as an appropriate actor in the public sphere of national politics. As Cindy Patton argues in her examination of recent gay rights discourse in the United States, "new-right identity is constructed through an asymmetry of knowledge and self-knowledge: occupying the hazardous space of being able to 'know it when you see it' while evading the charge that 'it takes one to know one.'"[34] The debates attempted, then, to locate male homosexuality firmly outside the walls of Parliament.

One of the few MPs who did not succumb to the discursive strategies employed in the debates and actively argued against the ways homosexuality was being constructed was Baroness Gaitskell, who asserted that "I personally do not regard homosexuality as a disease" and further pointed out "after all, not everything in the heterosexual garden is lovely" (Lords, 1965, 126, 127). "I do not believe that homosexual behaviour between consenting adults is harmful to the community," she declared, "or can have a serious effect on the whole moral fabric, as it is called, of social life. The whole moral fabric of social life often looks somewhat tattered to me after I have read my morning newspapers, or even my Sunday papers. The misdemeanors between man and woman far outnumber those between man and man" (128). Her voice, however, was generally drowned out by supporters as well as naysayers, eager to focus attention away from the instability of the heterosexual family cell and toward the pathological outsider, the homosexual.

Given the pathologizing discourse of the debates, then, what was the major issue that pushed the reforms through? Blackmail. Both the pro-reform and anti-reform speakers acknowledged that the legal punishments for those caught engaging in homosexual acts served as, in the words of several speakers, a "blackmailer's charter," a phrase first coined during the Oscar Wilde trial by Sir Travers Humphrey to refer to the Labouchère amendment of 1885 that criminalized all homosexual acts as "gross indecency." G. R. Strauss quoted the claim of the former attorney-general, Lord Jowitt, that "95 percent of blackmail cases that come before the court are concerned with homosexuality" (Commons, 1966, 805). Notably, some of the anti-reform speakers suggested that removing the legal punishments would barely lessen this problem: since homosexuality was still considered a wholly unacceptable "perversion" by many, blackmail could still be effective even if homosexual acts were legal. But the compelling argument seems to have been that the current laws criminalizing homosexuality only served to make these outsiders susceptible to blackmail — and thus made homosexuals, already seen by some as disloyal to the foundational tenets of the national body, a threat to national security as potential spies.

The perception of such a threat was based, in fact, on at least one real case: that of John Vassall, exposed as a spy for the Soviets in 1962. Vassall had been a spy for seven years, beginning while he had been a clerk in the British Embassy in Moscow and continuing after he was stationed back in London. His claim was that he was threatened with blackmail by the KGB unless he became a spy. The KGB did have photographs of him attending a party, set up by the embassy translator Sigmund Mikhailsky (known by the British to be a KGB plant but nonetheless tolerated), during which he participated in homosexual acts. But as Rebecca West suggests, it was quite possible that the party was staged by the KGB in order to give Vassall a protective excuse once he was caught.[35] Since Vassall was not highly closeted, and he was a very effective spy, this theory seems likely; and as West argues, he had far worse to look forward to were he found to be a spy than were he found to be gay. His case was read differently by different audiences: he was seen either as a typical example of the traitorous, disloyal homosexual, or he was evidence that the law had to be changed to help prevent blackmail of those who might have access to confidential information. The latter position seems to have won out.

Baroness Gaitskell, however, had a different take on the implications of the then-current law. Instead of focusing on the homosexual as a potential spy, she turned the argument around by noting that in their current system, each member of British society was expected to be an informer: "What kind of loyalty can we expect from these people towards a society which hounds them, often in such a humiliating way? What can be more squalid than the police spy in the public lavatory? No blame on the police officer, for he is carrying out his instructions. But what of the general public, the doctors, the psychologists, the priests—are they to be informers, too? The whole business of being an informer is most repulsive in a democracy" (Lords, 1965, 128–29). She explicitly connects "spy" and "informer," two terms that, I would argue, essentially describe the same subject despite their different usages. The implications of her argument are that the current legal structure ensures that everyone is set against each other in support of the nation/state; interpersonal disloyalty, then, is the groundwork for national security, a never-ending cycle of informers informing on potential informers. It is perhaps worth a reminder that "informer"—and "information," for that matter—come from "inform," which means "to shape." In this context, information shapes not only individual agency and subjectivity but also the nation/state itself.

Saving Ulster from Sodomy: Decriminalization in Northern Ireland

The debates in Britain laid the groundwork for a series of events that took place in Northern Ireland in the 1970s and early 1980s. The decriminalization of male homosexuality in Great Britain in 1967 was not extended to Northern Ireland; the very brief discussion of this possibility was sidelined with the claim, often repeated by the British government in the 1970s, that Northern Ireland was different from the rest of Great Britain, had different moral codes, and that an extension of the acts to Northern Ireland would thus be inappropriate. Later actions by the Northern Ireland police force, however, indicate that the British government was not, after all, practicing broad-minded cultural relativism or acknowledging Northern sovereignty when it left the laws criminalizing male homosexuality on the books.

In 1976, the Royal Ulster Constabulary (RUC) raided the homes of twenty-three gay men in Belfast, ostensibly because one of the men was trafficking in drugs; once inside, the RUC looked for evidence, based on information given by the parents of one of the younger men, that they were breaking the sodomy laws. The RUC used this opportunity to question thirteen of the men, officers and members of the Gay Liberation

Society (GLS) of Belfast, and to take papers, membership lists, and other documents associated with the society.

The reasons given for this assault were various. Of course, the drugs were the primary excuse; and to give the police some credit, they did find a small bag of marijuana. One RUC officer even made the claim that, by exposing members of the GLS, he was helping them "[lift] the burden of guilt and secrecy."[36] But these excuses aside, why the sudden interest in the GLS, the "gay libbers," as the RUC called them, when the group had been in operation for several years and when the sodomy laws were, prior to this point, so rarely enforced by the RUC? As one of the harassed gay men put it, "You'd think Mr. Rees [then secretary of state] would want to encourage it, wouldn't you? It's almost the only form of non-sectarian activity left."[37]

An article in the Northern Ireland Gay Rights Association (NIGRA) newsletter suggests one answer: the RUC was looking to thwart the potential for a dirty-tricks campaign against British government officials who opposed apartheid, a campaign to be launched by the South African Bureau of State Security (BOSS).[38] Were this the case, the British government would have been working in concert with security forces in Northern Ireland in order to protect the reputation of one of its members from being "accused" of homosexuality. By threatening Northern gay rights activists with the outing of their group's membership, the RUC would hope to prevent them from working with BOSS. In short, the state forces were hoping to use the threat of blackmail on the GLS to prevent GLS members from working with BOSS to blackmail government officials. But this begs the question, why would gay men work with BOSS to begin with? The RUC might have assumed that the gay rights activists were insufficiently loyal to the British government, an assumption certainly fueled by anti-gay discourse of the 1950s and 60s. Within this reading, homosexuals were treated like a revolutionary cell organized to undermine the British state.

But certainly the RUC wouldn't need the potential of a BOSS dirty-tricks campaign to find a reason to target the membership lists of the GLS. As late as 1994, more than a decade after decriminalization, there is evidence that the RUC swept gay male cruising spots in Northern Ireland, looking for informers.[39] As long as homosexual acts remained illegal, the RUC would have had an even easier time of it: to a closeted gay man, the possibility of legal proceedings and consequent outing was a particular threat and was an extra boon to an RUC eager to entrap possible informers. Although the leaders of the GLS were "out" in at least some public contexts, the membership lists presumably contained names of some who were not publicly recognized as homosexual and who were thus susceptible to blackmail. By threatening to expose members of one kind of "cell," then, the RUC hoped to gain assistance in penetrating other cells, particularly paramilitary groups. And given the discomfort with homosexuality historically expressed by those engaged in national struggles, finding a gay loyalist or republican paramilitary would presumably be a particularly welcome boon; such a person would likely be very susceptible to blackmail by the RUC. The very issue that facilitated decriminalization in Great Britain, in short, had the opposite effect in the North—because the North had an interest in state-sponsored blackmail.

Regardless of the reasons for the RUC sweep, it turned out to be an important catalyst for the gay rights movement. Jeff Dudgeon, an activist and one of those harassed by the police, used the incident to push legally for decriminalization to be extended to Northern Ireland. He did so by bringing the police abuse to the attention of the European Commission of Human Rights, and he asked for damages as well as a change in the law. He did not win the damages, but over the course of four years of trials, he did effect a change in the law in 1982.[40] Part of the reason he eventually succeeded is that the Standing Committee on Human Rights in Northern Ireland had already made its statement in support of the law changes, and the Labour government had already assured the commission that it planned to change the law.

But the changes to the law were postponed by the Labour government, already on shaky ground since the end of the Liberal/Labour pact and holding the government by a slim margin, because it wanted the support of Northern unionists. The secretary of state at the time, Roy Mason, claimed that the government was "hesitant to go ahead without the broad consent of the Northern Irish people in this 'sensitive and personal area'"—suggesting that the government had no right to intervene in personal affairs and thus, paradoxically, that it would continue to criminalize the personal affairs of gay men in Ulster.[41] During the submission period for the draft order, the Reverend Ian Paisley of the Democratic Unionist Party (DUP) began his "Save Ulster from Sodomy" campaign, working the issue through the pulpit and a petition drive. In his often-quoted sermon "How Roy Mason Is Pushing Ulster into the Cesspool of Sodomy," he warned that decriminalization would mean that God would let loose a plague of child molesters on the land—an interesting detail, particularly because at this time evidence suggests that he knew of a child molester by the name of William McGrath in his very own church, to be exposed in the Kincora affair a few years later.[42] His own "accurate" prophecies of child molestation, ostensibly tied to the decriminalization of homosexuality, were quite possibly dependent upon his own silence about (and thus, arguably, his complicity in a larger conspiracy of) child molestation that preceded the Dudgeon law reform case.

Although one might assume, particularly from the latter information, that the DUP might have a similar stake in decriminalization in order to prevent the British government from using information against its own members, it seems to have been willing to take the risk; as Paisley's treatment of Kincora suggests, individuals could always be excised and pilloried as aberrations, as foreign bodies in the DUP family cell. The "Save Ulster from Sodomy" campaign provided a way to establish Ulster's moral, social, and political independence from the rest of Great Britain. Britain's own changes in the law in the 1960s were cited as the reason that, in the words of DUP councillor George Graham, "England — that once great nation — had been brought down to the level it was today [because] of this sin, and because of debauchery" — an argument that drew on British anti-homosexual discourse from the Wilde trials onward. Alderman George Willey hoped that "'this little corner of the United Kingdom will manage to stave off the onslaught of people who sit at Westminster dreaming up ideas on law, the like of which we have before us tonight,'" and stated his sorrow that "they did not have a government at Stormont to deal with this matter."[43] The intended actions of Roy Mason, who eventually backed down from law reform, were seen as a case of "Direct Rule Decadence," in the words of the *Protestant Telegraph*.[44] Paisley referred to it as Mason's most "recent effort to destroy the moral fibre of Ulster."[45] Not surprisingly, homosexuality was generally described as a threat to the family, "the microcosm and vital basic unit of society" — more so, clearly, than divorce, which many in the North supported and which did come to pass during this time.[46] Homosexuality was also described in the *Protestant Telegraph* as a communist plot, something that revolutionary communists — like Henry Hay, founder of the homophile Mattachine Society — encouraged to dishearten a nation.[47]

Again, homosexuality is the foreign body par excellence: uncontainable, a plague and a communist plot, a threat from outside that serves to unite the Protestant Ulster nation in a claim to political sovereignty by safeguarding the family cell against British and communist decadence. The Catholic Church, of course, was somewhat stymied by this turn, not

'Righteousness exalteth a nation: but sin is a reproach to any people.'

(Proverbs 14 : 34)

The Secretary of State for Northern Ireland has announced that by the undemocratic system of Orders in Council he is going to legalise homosexuality — sodomy, in Northern Ireland. Such an action taken, without proper consultation with the Northern Ireland people, and, without proper full parliamentary procedure, not only constitutes a breach of constitutional rights, but, in such a matter of morals, an undermining of the moral fabric of Ulster.

There are many matters in Ulster which require immediate legislation, these Mr. Mason sweeps under the carpet but is prepared to legislate on a matter which can only bring God's curse down upon our people. **Sodomy is sin and should be repented of and not legislated for.**

The word of God says:—

"For this cause God gave them up unto vile affections: for even their women did change the natural use into that which is against nature: and likewise also the men, leaving the natural use of the woman, burned in their lust one toward another; men with men working that which is unseemly, and receiving in themselves that recompense of their error which was meet." (ROMANS 1 : 26 & 27)

"Who knowing the judgement of God, that they which commit such things are worthy of death, not only do the same, but have pleasure in them that do them." (ROMANS 1 : 32)

PETITION

To the Secretary of State for Northern Ireland, the Right Honourable Roy Mason, M.P.

We the undersigned being electors of Northern Ireland hereby declare our unalterable opposition to the implementation of the recommendation of the Standing Advisory Commission on Human Rights in respect of homosexuality or to any such change in the law of Northern Ireland relating to homosexuality. Further we fervently believe that no change in the law of Northern Ireland relating to homosexuality should be made without the consent of the electors of Northern Ireland.

I hereby solemnly declare and affirm that I am an elector of Northern Ireland, and that I have not previously signed this petition.

ELECTOR'S NAME	FULL ADDRESS

Please return to:
**THE PETITION ORGANISER,
1A AVA AVENUE, ORMEAU ROAD,
BELFAST BT7 3BN**

Printed petition forms can be obtained from the address below
Additional names can be attached to above form

ALL FORMS TO BE RETURNED BEFORE TUESDAY, 15th NOVEMBER, 1977
THIS PETITION IS ORGANISED BY THE ULSTER DEMOCRATIC UNIONIST PARTY AND SUPPORTED BY OTHER GROUPS THROUGHOUT ULSTER

DUP campaign against the decriminalization of homosexuality petition, 1977 at all eager to support the DUP but certainly not eager to decriminalize male homosexuality either—in this case, a very effective move on the part of Paisley. He appealed to a conviction in Northern Irish society that persists regardless of the religious affiliation of its adherents: that the family cell is vulnerable and must be safeguarded from "external" threat. The homosexual threat in this case is projected outside of Ulster and into decadent Great Britain; Irish nationalists and Ulster unionists can thus share resistance to this threat. Although the support for the campaign was far from universal, the DUP gathered almost seventy thousand signatures on its petition, and the British government cited the campaign's success as part of the evidence for a large-scale popular resistance to decriminalization in the North.[48]

The British government's resistance pushed Dudgeon to bring his case to the European Commission of Human Rights. His challenge struck at one of the DUP's assumptions: a limited and heteronormative definition of home, family, and the private sphere. The changes in the law for which he fought were effected by successfully appealing to Article 8 of the European Convention on Human Rights, which states that

> 1) Everyone has the right to respect for his private and family life, his home and his correspondence.
> 2) There shall be no interference by a public authority with the exercise of this right such as is in accordance with the law and is necessary in a democratic society in the interests of national security, public safety or the economic well-being of the country, for the prevention of disorder or crime, for the protection of the rights and freedoms of others.[49]

Dudgeon thus won on an appeal to the sanctity of privacy, despite the potential arguments that could have been made against his case in favor of retaining the laws for the sake of national security or the prevention of disorder or crime. Of course, the government could hardly respond by arguing that decriminalization would make it trickier to get informers. Dudgeon's victory was only a partial victory, however. He had tried to get the European court to recognize that he had been a victim of discrimination on the basis of sex, discrimination ostensibly proscribed by Article 14. Since they had ruled on Article 8, however, the court saw no need to consider the case under Article 14. Dudgeon's freedoms, therefore, were as a private person, rather than as a member of a class of persons.

There are two ways to see this victory. The most hopeful one for queer activists is, as I have suggested, to see it as a victory over a purely heterosexual definition of privacy—even though, significantly, the decision did nothing to redefine "home" and "family." Nonetheless, this is by no means a small victory. But one could also see this as pushing homosexuals more firmly back into the political closet. That is, by not ruling on Article 14, the freedoms gay men would enjoy would be *limited* to the private sphere, a marginalization that ensures that the public sphere remains the space in which heterosexuality, and only heterosexuality, is rightly performed. Privacy in this case, as I have suggested, becomes a cell of a different kind, one always implicit in the notion of the cell: a prison cell—a confined, limited, and limiting space. The "revolutionary cell" of the Gay Liberation Society was defanged; with private liaisons decriminalized, the perception of the need for further reform disappeared in the public imagination. Cross-community progressive political allegiances formed in this period atrophied, and in liberal circles a kind of political complacency returned. But the general public perception of homosexuality was unchanged; the public sphere, defined primarily by competing nationalist political positions (i.e., nationalist/republican versus unionist/loyalist), would remain, for a while at least, unchallenged by any further threats to its microcosmic mirror, the family cell.[50]

"An Irish Solution to an Irish Problem": Decriminalization in the Republic

Although the campaign for decriminalization in the Republic of Ireland took place over a longer period of time and sparked less concentrated public debate, the implications of the way in which it was resolved are no less significant than those attending Northern Irish law reform. In particular, the majority decision of the Supreme Court suggested that the Irish Constitution's construction of the state and family defines the "common good" to the exclusion of the public and private freedom of gay men.[51] Despite the many elements of his attack on the laws criminalizing male homosexuality, David Norris's eventual success, like Dudgeon's, rested solely on the extent to which the laws infringed upon his rights as a private person.

In the Republic, the campaign for equal rights for homosexuals was finally successful in 1993, but it actually began before the Dudgeon case was submitted. According to the Constitution, Ireland maintains prior (British) law except when explicitly repealed, so the Republic remained subject both to the 1861 Offences Against the Person Act and the 1885

Labouchère amendment. David Norris, a lecturer at Trinity College (later to become a senator in the Oireachtas), former chair of the Irish Gay Rights Movement, and member of both the Committee for Homosexual Law Reform and the National Gay Federation, actively campaigned for law reform from the early 1970s onward. In 1974, after working on behalf of gay men arrested under the 1867 and 1885 laws, Norris and others in the law reform movement decided to sue the State of Ireland for infringing on the civil and human rights of gay Irishmen. His primary argument was that the laws were unconstitutional: he maintained that the laws contradicted the Preamble of the Constitution, which speaks to the need for "due observance of prudence, justice and charity, so that the dignity and freedom of the individual may be assured," as well as Article 40, sections 1 and 3, in which citizens are said to be equal before the law and in which the state guarantees to respect and defend the rights of its citizens, respectively.[52] The right to which he was appealing in this instance was the right to privacy, established in an earlier case involving marital privacy and, as he argued, implied by the Preamble.[53] In the words of the report, Norris claimed that privacy "is a right which adheres to every citizen as such and which places a limit on the power of the State to control his personal conduct where neither the exigencies of the common good nor the protection of public order or morality necessitates such control."[54] Norris's appeal to privacy was modeled in part on the success of the Dudgeon case. His legal strategy, however, was not confined to the important but potentially limiting appeal to privacy. Like Dudgeon, he also claimed that gay men were inappropriately and unconstitutionally discriminated against on the basis of sex, since the laws were only applied to men. He appealed to the European Convention on Human Rights, to which Ireland was a signatory. And he objected to the law on the basis that it limited the right to assembly and free expression—a challenge to the notion that sexuality is primarily a private issue.

Norris's initial case failed, as did his appeal to the Supreme Court. The relationship of male homosexuality to religion and to marriage and family, institutions expressly addressed in the Constitution, was the main focus of attention and dissent in both cases. With regard to the former issue in the appeal, Chief Justice C. J. O'Higgins stated in the majority opinion that "on the ground of the Christian nature of our State and on the grounds that the deliberate practice of homosexuality is morally wrong, that it is damaging to the health both of individuals and the public and, finally, that it is potentially harmful to the institution of marriage, I can find no inconsistency with the Constitution in the laws which make such conduct criminal. It follows, in my view, that no right of privacy, as claimed by the plaintiff, can prevail against the operation of such criminal sanctions." "Homosexuality has always been condemned in Christian teaching as being morally wrong," he argued. "It has equally been regarded by society for many centuries as an offence against nature and a very serious crime." Since the Constitution defines Ireland as a Christian nation in the Preamble and in its invocation of God, legalizing homosexual practice, he argued, would be a challenge to that constitutional definition. Dissenting with this reading, Mr. Justice J. McCarthy suggested that the chief justice was defining Christianity in a very particular and limited way: "In so far as the judgment of Kenny J. in McGee's Case, in referring to the Christian and democratic nature of the State, is a relevant identification of source . . . I would respectfully dissent from such a proposition if it were to mean that, apart from the democratic nature of the State, the source of personal rights, unenumerated in the Constitution, is to be related to Christian theology, the subject of many diverse views and practices, rather than Christianity itself, the example of Christ and the great doctrine of charity which He preached. Jesus Christ proclaimed two great commandments — love of God and love of neighbour; St. Paul, the Apostle to the Gentiles, declared that of the great virtues, faith, hope and charity, the greatest of these is charity (1 Cor. 13, 13)." Mr. Justice Henchy further suggested that even in cases where the doctrinal issues were clear, as in the "seven deadly sins," "it would be neither constitutionally permissible nor otherwise desirable to seek by criminal sanctions to legislate their commission out of existence in all possible circumstances." Theirs, however, was the minority opinion.

The constitutional invocation of Christianity was not the only basis on which Norris's claims were rejected; the Constitution's protection of the family also led to legal wrangling. The justices were divided, for instance, about whether Norris could appeal to marital privacy as a basis for his claim that the proscriptions against sodomy were unconstitutional. Since he was an avowed homosexual, argued the chief justice, he would not marry and thus did not have the proper *locus standi* to challenge the law on those grounds. Mr. Justice J. McCarthy, however, believed that Norris could appeal to the invasion of marital privacy because, as he put it, "there have been many male homosexuals who were happily married — an obvious example in Irish history is Oscar Wilde whose conviction was under s. 11 of the Act of 1885." The logic supporting certain parts of the court's majority decision relating to marriage was similarly selective. According to the chief justice, "homosexual conduct can be inimical to marriage and is per se harmful to it as an institution." The justification for this claim is that "as long ago as 1957 the Wolfenden Committee acknowledged, in relation to Great Britain, the serious harm such conduct caused to marriage not only in turning men away from it as a partnership in life but also in breaking up existing marriages. That was the conclusion reached as to the state of facts before the criminal sanctions were removed. One can only suspect that, with the removal of such sanctions and with the encouragement thereby given to homosexual conduct, considerably more harm must have been caused in Great Britain to marriage as an institution." Chief Justice O'Higgins's reading of the report of the Wolfenden Committee, however, was deeply flawed. Although he was correct in asserting that Wolfenden acknowledges the threat of male homosexuality to marriage, the committee's conclusion was not that decriminalization would increase homosexual practice and therefore harm marriages. It did state that homosexual behavior on the part of men had been known to break up marriages or prevent men from marrying, and that they "deplored" such damage. It noted, however, that lesbian behavior and adultery would presumably have the same effect and were not subject to legal punishment. And it further submitted that legal and social prohibitions against homosexuality might encourage a homosexual man to marry a woman "simply for the sake of conformity with the accepted structure of society or in the hope of curing his condition"; such an act, it said, "may result in disaster."[55] In a blatant distortion of the Wolfenden Committee's findings, the justice's comments imply that a threat to marriage inheres in homosexuality itself, not in the sociopolitical and legal environment in which homosexuals find themselves.

The chief justice's statements do imply that homosexuality and by extension heterosexuality are not fixed identity constructs but rather patterns of desire and action that are subject to change. His comments make this clear, particularly when he asserted that "the homosexually orientated can be importuned into a homosexual lifestyle which can become habitual." Although seeing sexuality as a potentially unfixed set of behaviors is by no means a conservative position per se — in fact, it is one taken by many queer activists — the justice's statements make clear the political pitfalls of this approach to sexuality: as in the decriminalization debates in England in the 1960s, the justice treats homosexuality as a contagion that must be contained. Reinforcing this position, he argued that "male homosexual conduct has resulted, in other countries, in the spread of all forms of venereal disease and this has now become a significant public-health problem in England," although his claim has no factual support. It overlooks the fact that the gay activist community itself was directly responsible for raising overall AIDS awareness in Ireland and spearheading positive public health initiatives (Rose, 22–25), highlighting instead the discursive connection between homosexuality and "contagion," both literal and figurative. Chief Justice O'Higgins further stated that "exclusive homosexuality, whether the condition be congenital or acquired, can result in great distress and unhappiness for the individual and can lead to depression, despair and suicide," despite arguments presented in the original case suggesting that these negative behaviors do not come from homosexuality itself but are reactions to the social stigma attached to it, stigma only reinforced by its criminalization. The "concern" for the homosexual that somehow supports anti-homosexual legislation barely masks, I would argue, a concern about the instability of heterosexuality. Were the latter fixed and immutable, no legislation against the former would be necessary. In response to this fear of instability, the discourse that legally constructs male homosexuality offers only two ways of reading it: either homosexuality is a "congenital" condition, a disease; or it is a set of chosen acts, a contagion. Obviously, neither position offers gay men a particularly satisfying political subject-position.

By focusing on these two constructions, the majority opinion deflected attention from Norris's other claims: that the laws threatened his right to free expression and assembly. This claim was dismissed based on the fact that Norris himself had never been arrested despite his open avowal of his homosexuality. When the case came before the European Court of Human Rights, this part of the legal strategy was dropped; again, as I suggest with regard to the Dudgeon case, the practical implications are that the public sphere is to be preserved for the performance of heterosexuality. Even one of the Supreme Court justices who dissented from the majority opinion, Justice Henchy, tacitly reinforced the latter presumption when he stated that Norris's "public espousal of the cause of male homosexuals in this State may be thought to be tinged with a degree of that affected braggadocio which is said by some to distinguish a 'gay' from a mere homosexual." To be "gay," Henchy implied, is to move homosexuality from the contained private sphere to the public and to make one's difference from the heteronormative visible; such behavior, even when legal, is clearly objectionable.

The focus on privacy continued in the European courts. Norris, like Dudgeon, eventually won a judgment in the European Court of Human Rights on the grounds that the Irish law was in violation of the European Convention on Human Rights Article 8—that is, the right to privacy. The Dudgeon case provided the obvious precedent, since the laws on which the court was ruling were the same. Despite the court's ruling, it took another four years after the court's judgment for the Irish government to pursue a change in the law. The justices in the Supreme Court had noted firmly that Norris's references to the Convention were inconsequential; Ireland had never incorporated the Convention into its own law, a fact that might be seen as further evidence that it saw Europe as a threat to its sovereignty. But, as Rose points out, member states of the Council of Europe could be suspended or expelled for failing to implement rulings of the court. When it was eventually introduced, the legislation to decriminalize (with an equal age of consent) moved quickly through both houses, with the help of GLEN briefing documents.[56] As mentioned at the start of this chapter, the most vocal resistance came from Family Solidarity, whose members saw the European Court's ruling as "another example of Europe imposing its ethical values on Ireland" (as quoted in Rose, 47).

The law fully decriminalized male homosexual activity, going further than the British law insofar as it provided an equal age of consent and did not make exceptions for the military. David Norris addressed the Seanad in June of 1993 following the passage of the bill in the Dáil. Using GLEN's rhetorical strategy, outlined at the start of this chapter, Norris commended his colleagues in the Lower House:

> By effectively wiping the lingering shame of British imperial statute from the record of Irish law our colleagues in the Dáil have done a good days work. I confidently anticipate that we in this House will complete that work honourably. I have always said in defiance of comments from abroad that the Irish people were a generous, tolerant, compassionate and decent people and that this would one day be reflected even in that sensitive area of the law governing human sexuality. By enacting such a law in what is admittedly a delicate area we are extending the human freedoms of all citizens in this state. As the great apostle of Catholic emancipation Daniel O'Connell said in pleading his case at the bar of British public opinion, human dignity and freedom are not finite resources. By extending these freedoms to others one's own freedom is itself enhanced and not diminished. This is the kind of Irish solution to an Irish problem of which we as Irish men and women can feel justly proud.[57]

His repeated insistence here on the Irishness of the bill implies the pro-
tectionist background against which the law reformers had been working; the bill is framed as a defense against "comments from abroad"
rather than as a manifestation of a threat from abroad (i.e., Europe). This
is but one section of Norris's extensive and powerful speech in which he
outlined the history of Irish law reform and the arguments for and
against it. Throughout his speech, he systematically (and humorously)
struck at almost every challenge to homosexuality that has been presented over the years. At the end of the speech, however, he evoked the
one issue that still troubled the status of both gay men and lesbians:

> There is one other argument that I would like to address. I heard
> in the Lower House one member say that if this law were passed
> it would be the thin end of the wedge and he might have to wit-
> ness the horrible spectre of two men holding hands at a bus
> queue. May I say that if his mind were to be genuinely disturbed
> by such a prospect then his mental balance is precarious indeed.
> From the cradle I have been brainwashed with heterosexuality, I
> have frequently witnessed the spectacle of young heterosexual
> couples holding hands and enthusiastically kissing at those very
> same bus stops, and I merely wished them well and passed on
> my way. May I reassure the House that should two young men
> or two young women hold hands at a bus stop in Dublin the is-
> land will not be overwhelmed with earthquakes and turbulence,
> nor will the world come to an unexpected end. (23)

By mentioning that he had been "brainwashed with heterosexuality,"
Norris could be read as attempting to calm fears about the contagion of
homosexuality: if he was exposed to heterosexuality and remained homosexual, the reverse is likely to be true as well. But this section of the
speech also points to the "Irish problem" that remained: although gay
men were now allowed their private sexuality, public space was still
treacherous for both gay men and lesbians.

"Occupied Country": Nationalism, Feminism, and the Representation of Lesbianism

By including the hypothetical "two young women" in the remarks cited
above, Norris includes a group not specifically addressed by the anti-
homosexuality laws; given the legacy of British law, the term "homosexual" has applied legally to men, not women. Justice J. McCarthy,
in his dissenting opinion in the Supreme Court decision, stated that "it
is not appropriate to seek to make any comparable assessment of the

situation of the female homosexual—suffice it to say that no evidence was led at the trial in respect of such persons. From one's own knowledge of life in the Irish community, the situation of the female homosexual is not affected in any significant way either by the existence of the impugned sections or by contemporary mores." What "one's own knowledge" was is unclear from this section, but it is hard to believe that lesbians have been unaffected by "contemporary mores." In fact, lesbians have been part of the gay rights movement from the beginning, and they have also been part of the women's movement, which, as Rose has noted, inspired and provided political models for the gay rights movement. Lesbians have been active in these groups because they face containment both as queers and as women. That containment, I suggest, has come not only from within nationalist discourses.

The absence of lesbianism from much public discourse has been both a blessing and a curse: a blessing, of course, insofar as lesbianism per se has not been subject to legal prohibitions. But, of course, lesbians are women, and women have been subject to regulation through the family cell. Lesbianism, both as an identity and a practice, has been seen as part of a larger movement of asserting women's rights and has often been conflated with feminism—perhaps most notably in Great Britain in 1921, when a bill was introduced into Parliament to extend the Labouchère amendment to apply to "acts of gross indecency by females."[58] Weeks suggests that Arabella Kennealy's 1920 text, *Feminism and Sex Extinction*, may have influenced the debates; she saw feminism as a threat to the family and, in particular, parenthood, because it turned women away from reproduction and toward "masculinism," behavior in turn increasingly, but not exclusively, linked with lesbianism. These beliefs were echoed in the debates in Commons. Weeks notes that the bill was dropped for two reasons: one, the "liberal" view that lesbianism was a sickness—that is, the same view adopted toward male homosexuality in later decriminalization debates—and two, the view that criminalizing lesbian acts would actually alert the female populace to practices of which they had never heard, and that such practices might then, as Weeks put it, "spread like a contagion" (107). The disease/contagion theory of lesbianism, like that of male homosexuality, was thus present but submerged by the belief that the practice was limited to a few. As Laura Doan argues, the popular image of the lesbian was just forming in this period and was not yet the focus of the kind of "moral panic" evoked by male homosexuality.[59] Anxieties were directed more toward feminism, the larger movement that had the potential to articulate alternatives to entrapment within the family cell and that seemed the bigger threat; but the fact that lesbians were newly visible members of that group sometimes made them easy targets of anti-feminist politics.[60] The responses to the linking of feminism and lesbianism within the feminist movement have been various, ranging from celebration to denial and exclusion. The latter response, I would argue, follows the same pattern and strategy as nationalist discourse. By accepting the logic of nationalism, feminists can do to lesbianism what nationalism has historically done to feminism: silence it in the name of "freedom," thus assisting the uncomplicated perpetuation of the family cell and the nationalist discourses that rest upon it.

To understand the relationship of Irish feminism to lesbianism, we must first examine the relationship between feminism and nationalism. Margaret Ward has argued that Irish feminist women's "emotional and ideological identification with nationalism, which always overrode all other considerations, was a crucial factor in preventing them from ever developing a strategy which could have encompassed a larger definition of liberation."[61] This is an oversimplification of the varieties of Irish feminism, certainly; but it is true that a large and active segment of Irish feminism has championed the cause of Irish liberation from English rule. The connection between feminism and nationalism has a long history, a history that begins at least as early as the nineteenth century and continues to the present day.[62] The connection between feminism and nationalism is hardly surprising: both feminism and Irish nationalism share a telos of "liberation," or emancipation from the oppressive hegemony (the colonial power structure, the patriarchy, etc.).

But herein also lies the bind of the feminist-nationalist alliance: women's movements are read through the "master narrative" of liberation, one that puts nationalism at the forefront as the more universally desirable telos. This hierarchy of concerns—national freedom over women's freedom—will be familiar to anyone who has studied the interrelationship of gender and nationalism. As Anne McClintock notes in her discussion of the ANC and Afrikaner nationalism, "too frequently, male nationalists have condemned feminism as divisive, bidding women hold their tongues until after the revolution."[63] The same has been argued of Marxism by such feminist writers as Simone de Beauvoir and Monique Wittig.[64] David Lloyd has persuasively argued that "the desire of nationalism is to saturate the field of subject-formation" and subordinate other emancipatory movements; its logic is that of the state, insofar as nationalism strives toward achieving the formation of a nation-state. Feminism, along with other movements such as labor unionism, may share an emancipatory logic with nationalism, but eventually as nationalism achieves its ends — the formation of the nation-state — the state must expunge those "cultural or social forms that are in excess of its own rationality and whose rationale is other than its own."[65] Feminism is one of those forms. But it is not, as Lloyd seems to imply, only the state-oriented trajectory of nationalism that leads to its subordination of feminism in particular. Feminism is already subordinated in a hierarchy based on a culturally constructed gender duality that sees women and women's concerns as secondary, as Other to the "universal" male subject. Nationalism, in short, cannot effectively contain a critique of gender oppression because it relies on that gender binary for its logic.

Further undermining the feminist potential within Irish nationalism, Irish nationalist iconography has consistently employed an image of a passive Virgin/Mother Ireland as the inspiration for its action. She becomes the body acted upon as well as acted for. June Levine writes in *Sisters*, her history of Irish feminism, that "the whole world, for women, was occupied country."[66] Artist Pauline Cummins reinforces this idea when saying that "as a woman my body was my country."[67] Though both feminist artists exploit the terminology of Irish national liberation — the need to get the "country" back from the colonizer — to point to the need for women's liberation, their choice of words shows, and arguably reinforces, the terms of the struggle. The desire to get the land back has been written as a male desire, and women have been written as the object of that desire by their metaphorization as the land itself. Within this system of desire and representation, women are perpetually locked in a passive position; they are the country that men occupy. Cummins's and Levine's rhetorical strategies show the extent to which the "public" language of nationalism has dominated public debate: to talk about women as women, rather than as metaphors for nation ("occupied country"), has encouraged the dismissal of feminism under the rubric of private concerns. To accept this state of affairs, however, is to accept the way in which nationalism defines and neutralizes feminism. The pattern of subordination and exclusion has been internalized by many feminists, however, and has been replicated in the subordination of lesbian concerns to feminist concerns. This subordination is based on those same constructions of "legitimate" public discourse that both allowed colonialism to flourish and have allowed nationalism to silence and marginalize feminism.

A variety of texts offer examples of the ways in which feminist writers have accepted these discursive patterns. Gifford Lewis's biography, *Eva Gore-Booth and Esther Roper*, offers a history of these early-twentieth-century feminists in which the possibility of lesbianism is negotiated with discomfort. It is worth noting here that Eva Gore-Booth is perhaps best known through Yeats's poem "In Memory of Eva Gore-Booth and Con Markievicz":

> I know not what the younger dreams —
> Some vague Utopia — and she seems,
> When withered old and skeleton-gaunt,
> An image of such politics.
> (*Poems*, 233-34, ll. 10-13)

Even lesbian writer and critic Emma Donoghue begins her important and insightful study of Eva Gore-Booth's poetry with the statement that "a couple of years ago all I knew of Eva Gore-Booth . . . was that she was one of the two sisters in the W. B. Yeats poem my mother used to quote."[68] Con Markievicz is best known as an Irish nationalist, the founder of the nationalist boy's group Fianna Éireann, member of Inghinidhe na hÉireann, and officer of the Irish Citizen Army. Eva Gore-Booth was a pacifist devoted to the causes of women's suffrage and trade unionism. Yeats, however, by writing his poetic description of Gore-Booth directly following that of Con Markievicz, lets Gore-Booth's politics be subsumed into Markievicz's militant nationalism in the poem; the "vague Utopia" and "such politics" could as easily refer to militant physical-force nationalism as to feminism or trade unionism. The end of the poem implies Anglo-Irish complicity in the rhetorical and artistic constructions that inspired the new Irish state ("We the great gazebo built / They convicted us of guilt"), further subsuming Gore-Booth's complex politics into the "larger" concerns of nationalism. Lewis's biography extracts Gore-Booth and her narrative from the containment of Yeats's poem, only to contain her further with respect to sexuality.

In her introduction to the lives of Gore-Booth and Esther Roper, Lewis addresses the issue of sexuality: "They were fortunate in living at a time when ladies could still set up home together in perfect equanimity with no suspicion of the dark wastes of psychopathology into which they had strayed" (2). Most of Lewis's introduction is devoted to the ways in which these women have been remembered and represented. But Lewis is clearly invested in excluding their relationship from the realm of the lesbian. She argues that "it would be wrong to assume that all pairs of women were lesbian; when they were they took very little trouble to conceal it, like Katherine Bradley and Edith Cooper, ecstatically ignorant of Freud. . . . Women, married and single, who might incline to physical affairs with other women actually did so if the opportunity presented itself; others didn't incline, and though women might form pairs this does not infallibly indicate a desire for lesbian love" (8). Lewis presumably defines lesbian love exclusively in terms of the genital sexual acts associated with it; Gore-Booth and Roper, devoted to transcendence of the physical, clearly do not fit this rather narrow definition. She adds: "Some female pairings were quite formal: . . . Eva Gore-Booth and Esther Roper never entered each other's bedrooms except in illness" (8).

That Lewis chooses to begin the biography this way suggests a strong investment in maintaining, to borrow Casement biographer Reid's term, the "purity" of her subjects. Lewis's assertion that women who wanted physical connections with other women invariably had them is a generalization one certainly cannot make today, and her assertion that their relationship was strictly "formal" presumes much. But more important, Lewis's treatment of the couple's sexuality forecloses any discussion of its importance for lesbian visibility. By relegating their relationship to the realm of the "merely" personal, Lewis refuses to recognize that their choice to live and love together was a personal choice with important political implications. As Emma Donoghue has written, "Whether Eva and Esther were celibate and calm in their feelings, celibate but impassioned, occasionally sexual, sexual early on and then 'transcending' it, or discreetly sexual right through their relationship, the fact of their lifelong lesbian partnership remains" (40). And that partnership was, to use Sheila Jeffreys's words, part of "a passionate commitment to women, a culture, a political alternative to the basic institution of male supremacy" that both characterizes these particular women's lives and lesbian feminism in general.[69] By drawing the boundary around lesbianism, however, Lewis allows feminism to monopolize the field of political possibilities at the expense of lesbian politics. Lesbianism is declared outside the realm of possibility from the very first chapter, which "frees" the narrative to deal with certainties and less controversial biographical topics. Whether or not this move represents the author's homophobia, it seems at least structured to sidestep the potential homophobia of readers — readers who presumably do not need feminism or trade unionism similarly explained away.

The discomfort with and erasure of lesbianism in the name of feminism is certainly not limited to biographical texts; similar strategies can be found at work in feminist fiction. Edna O'Brien's *The High Road* and Levine's *A Season of Weddings* demonstrate the subsumption of sexual politics by more "general" narratives. Though both writers begin to articulate the importance of lesbianism for their protagonists, both slip into a more comfortable narrative of self-discovery that silences the lesbian experience both of the protagonists and of the women they desire.

In *The High Road,* memories of a painful, unfulfilling heterosexual affair drive Anna, the narrator, to a Spanish town that borders the Mediterranean. She meets others also running from painful memories, most of which can be traced to heterosexual relationships or their ensuing familial instabilities. When the narrator is at the point of suicide, both from reliving her own past and from confronting others' pasts, she is saved by the attentions of Catalina, a local woman working for the hotel. Their friendship develops into a more intense affair. After the women share a night of physical love, Anna prepares to leave town. Her happy sense of interpersonal connection is disrupted first by the graffiti "lesbos" scrawled on Catalina's house and then, more tragically, with Catalina's murder by her husband. The narrative ends with Anna's preparations to leave the country, never to return.

The High Road evokes a powerful angst of disconnectedness, heightened by the pain of exile from familiar surroundings. At the point in the text at which Anna's isolation seems the most acute, however, the narrative hints at the possibility of interpersonal connection through an emerging recognition of repressed sexuality. Catalina brings Anna flowers, and that night she has a dream:

> I dreamed of rings. An entire room covered from floor to ceiling with them—throbbing, darting, as if they were lizards; had pulse, had life. . . . There were stones too, stones from the seashore. . . . I wanted to touch them, lick them. In the dream I am obliged to pick my favorite ring, and though tempted by many, by such luster, by such gleam and gleamings, I pick a gray-green stone with half its color drained, a forgotten stone such as might be dredged from the bottom of the sea or the bowels of the earth and left to molder, and as I picked it I thought, even within the dream, that it was a precursor of things to come. (56)

The dream, with its throbbing and tempting rings, suggests sexuality; Anna's choice of the "forgotten" stone brought up from the depths seems to indicate an acknowledgment of repressed homosexual desire, especially given that, later in the novel, Anna remembers an uncompleted sexual encounter with a "dusky girl" in London.[70]

This movement toward sexual self-recognition is reinforced by the next chapter, in which Anna sees Catalina again. When they finally consummate their love, however, the description of the connection, however clearly physical, is ambiguous:

> Then I felt the thwack of her arms around me and the clasp of her hands, and I stretched out and cleaved to her, through her opening to life; arms, limbs, torsos joined as if in an androgynous sculpture, the bloods going up and down merrily, two bloods, like mercury in a heated thermometer, even the cheeks letting go of all their scream and all their grumble and their thousand unspent kisses; tenderness, rabidness; hunger; back, back in time to that wandering milky watery bliss, infinitely safe like wine inside a skin or sap inside a tree, floating, afloat; boundaries burst, bursting, the mind as much as the body borne along, to this other landscape that was familiar yet unfamiliar, like entering a picture, a fresco, slipping through a wall of flesh, eclipsed inside the womb of the world, and throughout it all, her words, faint, sweet as vapor. (186)

The moment of physical connection is written as a kind of return to the womb, a reconnection to the Ur-Mother that works against the prior disconnectedness the narrator feels. This connection is not explicitly about sex, however; it is described as "the invisible sustenance, not what we sought from men, something other-womanly, primordial" (185). In the same vein, Anna describes the women of the area as having "an uncanny earthiness as if the high-heeled shoes that they wore were merely plinths which connected them to the earth beneath, not just its surface but to the foundations where the sewer and the sap flowed, way way beneath to the earth's root" (92). As in the "sex" scene, the Spanish women are written as primordial, earthy landscapes toward which desire travels.

In O'Brien's scheme, the connection between the two women works against the pain and lack of fulfillment that women get from their other relationships. Its reliance on an essentialist notion of women as earthy and fertile mothers not "seeking in each other what they seek in men," however, encourages us to read the sequence as something other than sexual. And it is worth noting here that Anna herself does not or cannot name this desire. Only afterward, when the graffiti aggressively names the act, do we have a kind of confirmation of what has happened. Through the graffiti, the narrative gives us a difficult and limited choice: confirm or deny the accusing scrawl, "lesbos." The ambivalence of the "sex" sequence gives us the opportunity to deny the scrawl, to plead a kind of innocence on the narrator's behalf; the narrator's own silence about the scrawl reinforces that presumption of "innocence." In other words, the narrative allows the reader to accept the homophobia of the community, to allow "lesbos" to remain a curse, even to be homophobic oneself while still sympathizing with the narrator. Even Catalina's murder does not require a critique of homophobia: she is killed by a jealous husband. Any specific criticism of homophobia is subsumed under the larger rubric of pain, alienation, and the impossibility of sustainable human connection.

O'Brien and Levine approach their texts from a different set of biographical circumstances. Levine is a self-described feminist with a firm commitment to supporting women's right to choose, to allowing people to name and practice their "self-determined sexuality" (*Sisters*, 295), and to challenging the uneven power relationship occasioned by heterosexual marriage, particularly as legally defined in Ireland. Edna O'Brien, on the other hand, does not openly identify herself as a feminist and has chosen to exile herself to England, a choice she discusses in some detail in *Mother Ireland*. June Levine's *A Season of Weddings* is a more self-conscious exploration of the politics of gender, class, and nationality. But the novels share disturbing similarities. *A Season of Weddings*, like *The High Road*, features a woman going to another country to escape an unfulfilling heterosexual relationship. The protagonist, Nora, uses the wedding of a friend's child as an excuse to get some distance on her troubled, sexless marriage. Her visit to India and consequent exposure to another culture provide her with different models of relationships, marriage, family—and sexism. Each culture has its traditions of female oppression, and both Nora and the mother of the bride, Maya, provide insights into the other's culture. As the story progresses, so too does Nora's friendship with Maya. But like *The High Road*, the sexual connection between the two women is never given a name and is only hinted at with professions of love, the occasional stroking of a face, and the sharing of a bed. At one point, however, Nora is forced to consider her own sexuality, and by implication her own homophobia, when she confronts her suspicion that her husband is gay. Nora ponders whether her decision to marry Dennis was subconsciously because of her own bisexuality. Maya responds, "A person is the way she is. Sometimes we cannot be that way. We have to do one way and smother another. Wimmen . . . have not the choices. And always, we must try to include, not destroy."[71] While never wholly endorsing Maya's philosophy, Levine nonetheless gives it the nod by never presenting a coherent counterargument. The suggestion that women must literally be self-sacrificing is challenged through Nora's horror at the practice of sati. But the choice to put up with sometimes stifling sexist traditions, to persist quietly, is not so easily challenged.

A Season of Weddings confronts the issue of sexuality much more directly than *The High Road*. Nora does not simply put her relationship behind her. She begins to accept "[the feelings] that had often stirred in her through the years" with "gentle waves of relief" (284). She recognizes that her choice to marry was possibly an alibi, and that "she felt incapable of slipping back into the old life" (285). Nonetheless, this novel shares with *The High Road* a silence about the love that dare not speak its name. In this case, the silence might be read as strategic: Levine's *Sisters* acknowledges that the claims that feminists were "unfeminine," "lesbians," and "harlots" plagued the 1970s Irish feminist movement (121). But the choice not to respond, to remain silent, is a capitulation, deliberate or not, to those who silence, contain, and oppress.

The two novels share other elements. The lesbian relationships in both novels take place in the realm of the non-Irish cultural Other. Though the texts attempt to write the women who have the relationships as allies in resistance to a patriarchal system of oppression, they also conveniently place lesbianism outside the realm of Irishness, potentially reinforcing the very discourse of foreignness applied so often to male homosexuality. And conveniently for the mainstream feminist master-narrative, the non-Irish lesbian Other in the story either remains behind or dies. She becomes part of the subplot, the larger plot being the awakening of one character's consciousness. In the case of *The High Road*, the narrator recognizes the general human condition of disconnectedness; in *A Season of Weddings*, the protagonist recognizes her own personal need for growth and self-recognition in the face of a patriarchal culture. Neither, however, returns explicitly to the relationship or desires that inspired such epiphanies.

This analysis is not meant to suggest that every literary text written by a feminist should include and celebrate lesbianism, or even that literature should have a political goal. But these texts are examples, symptoms of the internalization of what patriarchal discourse deems "appropriate," even in the private sphere. And they suggest the difficulty of exploring alternatives to containment — even in a purely imaginative space.

"We *Are* Home": ILGO and the Public Sphere

What spaces are available, then, for queers? Is there a way to "imagine the world otherwise," in the words of Ailbhe Smyth, to challenge the ways that lesbians and gays are contained by a nationalist discourse dependent upon the family cell?[72] These questions do not face only queers in the Republic of Ireland and Northern Ireland. Where queers fit, what their relationship is to the public and private spheres, are issues faced by many — including gays and lesbians of Irish descent across the Atlantic. In the early 1990s, while David Norris was still in court, another legal controversy was brewing: whether the Irish Lesbian and Gay Organization would be allowed to march in the St. Patrick's Day parade in New York City.[73] At issue was, and continues to be, the literal and figurative place of homosexuality and its relationship to Irish national identity. Since the controversy began when ILGO, a group with visible female leadership, made their request to march, the terms of the debate notably have not been limited to male homosexuality, although the response to the group as a whole has been remarkably similar to prior legal and cultural responses to male homosexuals who have entered the contentious waters of the public sphere.

ILGO's presence at the parade has been hotly contested by the Ancient Order of Hibernians (AOH), which, since it was given a permit for the parade "in perpetuity" in 1994, officially "owns" the parade.[74] Other Irish Americans and parade-goers of all ethnicities have also expressed their opinions about the parade controversy over the years. In a documentary called *Forever Fierce and Outta Control,* one of ILGO's videographers, Cecilia Dougherty, captured both the 1996 pre-parade protest march and the afternoon "Rock the Blocks" protests that ILGO had organized with other sympathetic organizations. At one point, the video captures a crowd of male onlookers shouting "queers go home" at the ILGO members and supporters. The latter respond with an even louder "we *are* home." The exchange resonates with a number of issues already raised in this chapter; in particular, it suggests the extent to which the "place" of homosexuality remains a contested issue. The controversy suggests that, both in American and Irish American constructions of identity and public space, homosexuality must be located elsewhere.[75]

What might it mean to say "queers go home," and what could the response "we *are* home" mean? The first impression one might get from the chant "queers go home" is that they meant "home" in the most literal and local sense: go back to your houses; get off the street; you queers are not welcome here, out in public. This could be read as an aggressive variation on the feelings Norris cites as coming from a member of the Dáil: even if homosexual practice is legal, no aspect of it should be visible. Despite the fact that no ILGO members were copulating in public, queer identity was and is seen by many as a verbal expression of one's preference for performing certain sexual acts. To express queer identity on St. Patrick's Day is thus considered inappropriate; it reminds one of sex, and sex is reserved for "home," or private space. As I was asked several times when I participated in the afternoon protests in 1997, why here? Why gay and lesbian identity in the St. Patrick's Day parade, of all places? Why not express this identity in private?

The answer is that the St. Patrick's Day Parade is a public space in which Irish identity is expressed, celebrated, and, in this case, contested. As Helena Mulkerns of *Hot Press Magazine* noted in 1995, echoing ILGO's own press statements and flyers: "It is interesting that New York's first official St Patrick's Day parade in 1762 was organised by Irish Protestants and Catholics as a protest to fight just such 'ancient hatreds'—the ethnic and religious discrimination that was rampant against Irish people living there. ILGO's statement on February 21st [1995] pointed out that 'Lesbians and gay men of all races and ethnicities now insist on that same simple right: participation in the life of our ethnic communities on equal terms with everyone else. It's ironic that in the 1990s the parade organisers discriminate against Irish people on the basis of sexual orientation.'"[76] Kieran Rose observes that "what was at issue was who would define what it is to be Irish" (32). To extend the irony Mulkerns mentions: many people, both in the film of the 1996 march and in the 1997 march in which I participated, saw the St. Patrick's Day parade as a specifically religious celebration, and a specifically Catholic one at that; this, for many onlookers, justified discrimination on the basis of sexual orientation. Historically, as Mulkerns suggests, it is inaccurate to see the St. Patrick's Day parade as a religious celebration, and by no means are all of the participants or perhaps even a majority of the onlookers Catholic. The parade itself, however, has become increasingly Roman Catholic over the years. In the video *Rock the Sham*, ILGO's cofounder and frequent spokesperson Anne Maguire expressed frustration that the legal rulings allow the Ancient Order of Hibernians "ownership" of the parade, effectively making this public spectacle a private Catholic affair, so the organization can discriminate against whomever it wishes.[77]

The United States does allow political parades in this country as part of the First Amendment right to free speech. But it is also ironic, given the history of the parade, that one of Mayor Rudolph Giuliani's oft-repeated justifications for excluding ILGO in 1997 was that the New York St. Patrick's Day parade was "not political"—ironic given that martial music is played by police and military organizations; that politicians march to be seen by their constituents; that NORAID, an American organization that funds the republican struggle in Northern Ireland, is allowed to march under its own banner, as are Friends of Irish Freedom. But these are unmarked, unremarkable parts of the parade. They are taken for granted and are thus not "political" in the popular sense of being contested at that time and place: they are undeniably Irish, and Irish is not political on St. Patrick's Day, regardless of the explicit political affiliations expressed by those marching. Unless, of course, one is Irish and gay or lesbian. This points, then, to a kind of paradox: homosexuality is private, homosexuality is political. ILGO's contestation of the parade thus brings to the foreground the inseparability of private and public or political. It exposes the falsehood of the claim, both popular and legal, that these spheres are and should remain separate.

As Lauren Berlant has persuasively suggested, in the United States, projections of the fantasy of the normal heterosexual family as an image of the nation, and repeated articulations and images of the assault on that image, take the place of the public sphere.[78] The difference between Ireland and the United States is that in Ireland the conflation of home, family, and nation is explicit; private and public are rhetorically intertwined in the Irish Constitution. But the United States legal structure has effected the same result through its manipulation of the right to "privacy"—a welcome protection for many individuals, but one that is based on the core assumptions that the private sphere is properly heterosexual. Although the U.S. Supreme Court finally struck down same-sex anti-sodomy laws in June of 2003, the Defense of Marriage Act (1996), ensuring that the U.S. federal government does not have to recognize homosexual marriages performed legally in its member states, remains in effect and exposes the complicity of the state in fixing the heterosexual family as the ideal private structure. The private is only selectively protected, then; the "home" and the private sphere to which queers are supposed to go, according to the jeering crowd, effectively do not exist for queers. Nor does the public sphere. The right to public expression, or "free speech," is similarly protected only selectively. A case in point: ILGO requested a permit for permission to march in a separate parade, one that would end before the official AOH parade would begin. It was denied by the city, however, because the latter claimed it could not protect ILGO from gay bashers or from the AOH. Legally speaking, protecting the city from traffic congestion received a higher priority than ILGO's right to free speech.

There is another, more subtle interpretation of the chant of "queers go home." Perhaps the most visible of the organizers, Anne Maguire and Marie Honan, are Irish nationals. They speak with Irish accents. They have been on television and radio repeatedly. So "go home" in this context, oddly enough, could mean "go back to Ireland"; it is an expression of the desire to exclude ILGO from Irish identity in the United States. This desire extends beyond the parade: during the gatherings in support of the release of republican prisoner Roisin McAliskey in 1995, Maguire and Honan, two women who are republican in sentiment, were accused by other Irish nationalists of being "traitors and British spies."[79] The rhetoric of disloyalty to the nation resonating throughout twentieth-century representations of homosexuals finds new life when Irish identity is expressed abroad, when nationalists are distant from the safe "home" of Ireland.

This phenomenon of exclusion becomes less strange when examined more closely: the AOH response to ILGO is an attempt to legitimize a certain narrative of Irish identity in the United States, one based on a history of conservative Irish Catholicism, patriarchy, and, of course, heterosexuality. The conservatism of Irish American Irish nationalists is closely tied to an investment in a simplified narrative of Irish history, in the absence of a simple spatial claim to identity: that is, if one does not reside within the spatial boundaries of Ireland, one needs an airtight narrative of descent that serves to protect the boundaries of group identity. Self-policing the borders of the Irish American community is deemed essential to control the fickle American public perceptions of a group that has historically been both demonized as nonwhite and, more recently, celebrated as Ur-white. Expanding the possibilities of who can be Irish blurs the distinction between (Irish) self and other; to include a category of people so consistently alienated as homosexuals is risky and destabilizing indeed. ILGO has posed such a threat, particularly because sexuality is so often an un(re)markable category: to accept ILGO means accepting the possibility that members of ILGO already exist within the sanctioned confines of the parade and of "Irishness." To deny ILGO access, to assert that their "home" is elsewhere, is implicitly to assert that gay men do not exist in the AOH; that no women who came to work in New York, Boston, and Philadelphia in the nineteenth century were lesbians; that no Irish-American priests or nuns are gay or lesbian; that the whole history of Irish emigration to the United States is not already inextricably bound up with gay and lesbian history. ILGO is an "otherable" group, conveniently enough, and by excluding it physically from the parade, the AOH as well as the crowd of hostile onlookers expressed a hope to exclude the people it represents from the narratives of Irish, Irish-American, and American identities. As the population of the United States becomes more complex and diverse, both in terms of the cultural and ethnic makeup of its inhabitants and the varieties of expression of politics, home, family, and individual identity, many Irish-Americans are pressured to conform to this fantasy of the ideal heterosexual family—the family cell—in order to be seen as normative, to maintain the hard-won status of "typical."

But this requires policing the public representations of Irishness. Anne Maguire has noted that the legitimization of Gay Pride Day can be seen as a strategy to facilitate the alienation of lesbians and gays from other aspects of public life: "Mayor Giuliani has basically told us 'you have your day in June,' referring to the Gay Pride Parade, which is all about containment. He doesn't seem to understand that we are lesbians and gay men of all ethnic and racial identities, not for one designated day in June, but for the other 364 days of the year as well."[80] As the "Frequently Asked Questions" portion of the official ILGO Web site stated, "as Irish lesbians and gay men, our cultural heritage and sexual identity are inseparably linked—we are Irish and gay."[81]

For the AOH, however, to be gay seems to imply one's citizenship in "an alternative sexual world," to quote Reid. One of the ways in which the AOH has justified its position about excluding ILGO is through the claim that, since over the years ILGO has been supported by queer activist groups from a range of nations and cultures, they are not *specifically* Irish. Support from the international gay and lesbian community, the participation of non-Irish groups such as the South Asian Lesbian and Gay Association, Las Buenas Amigas, and Jewish Activist Lesbians and Gays—all point to the queer as opposed to Irish loyalties of ILGO. In short, Irish is "home," whereas queer is "foreign"; they are mutually exclusive categories. This is no less true in the United States than it is in Ireland. In both places, Irishness needs to be protected from foreign threat.

There are encouraging signs in New York, however, just as there are in Ireland. When I participated in the parade in 1997, in the afternoon after the morning protests, I stood with a colleague, with an ILGO sign, and fielded questions and comments from the parade spectators. We did experience others' hostility, but also honest questions, and some productive discussions ensued with those who approached us. Overwhelmingly, we felt as if ILGO had become a part of the parade, and some people, even those not particularly sympathetic to ILGO, seemed disappointed that they did not see more ILGO members on the streets. In other words, ILGO is not included in any legal sense, but in the imagination of the public ILGO has become a part of this event. In 2002—a particularly charged year for the New York parade, since it was dedicated to those who died in the World Trade Center disaster—Mayor Michael Bloomberg invited ILGO to a breakfast on St. Patrick's Day. Aine Duggan of ILGO did not, however, suggest that this breakfast was a substitute for marching: "We're hoping that we can continue meeting with the mayor's office to ensure that the 2003 parade will be inclusive, just like this breakfast is inclusive today. And as you can see, we're all mingling here together, it's a very happy occasion, there's no controversy. It is possible for all Irish people to be in the same room at the same time and represent different interests."[82] ILGO's consistent commitment to the issue has meant that they have begun to claim a space in a public sphere under threat. All over the world, but particularly in New York, and particularly given the rhetoric of containment circulating after the attacks on the United States on September 11, 2001, it is all the more essential that such a sphere remain alive and vibrant.

In closing, I would like to return to the Republic of Ireland. Things have changed for the better since decriminalization. Irish queers have experienced at least accommodation, and occasionally active solicitation, by the mainstream. Starting in 1998, for instance, the lord mayor of Dublin began hosting a reception for the organizers of Gay Pride, and the city hung pride banners around town. I would argue, however, that these changes have come less because of the "traditional Irish values" embodied by nationalism than because of the "Celtic Tiger," that economic boom that began in the mid-1990s. Rocked by political crises in the 1980s and early 1990s centered on the instability of the family cell—particularly revelations about incest, abortion, child sexual abuse, and political complacency about them—the Republic of Ireland could breathe a sigh of relief when the Celtic Tiger provided a strong foothold in the European economy. Formerly an outsider, Ireland took center stage, and fears that Ireland would be damaged by the tide of "moral decadence from Europe" were lessened in the face of seeming economic prosper-

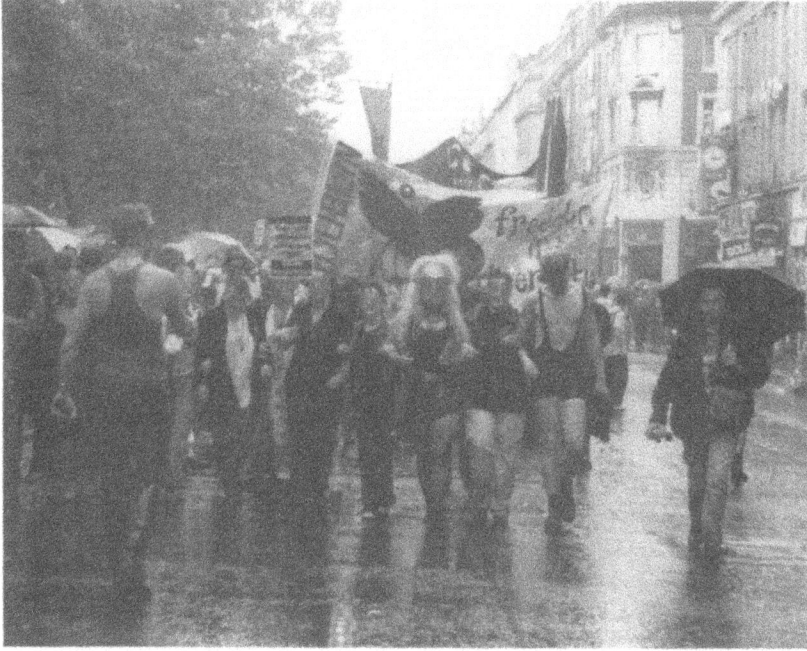

Gay Pride Parade, Dublin, 1998 (photo by author)

ity. Middle-class queers, then, were courted as economic animals, encouraged to spend their money in Ireland, even to return from emigration; their money would help to strengthen the nation.

But Ireland isn't always so liberal as its laws suggest, as we were reminded when Philadelphia gay writer Robert Drake was beaten into a brain-damaging coma by two Sligo men in his Sligo house just a few years ago. The Irish Constitution still protects the family as the "fundamental unit group of society." And queers in the North, where nationalist discourses clash, remain besieged, confined, and at risk. The improvement in the comfort of queers in Ireland, it seems, is contingent upon the belief that the opening of borders is an economic boon, not a threat—particularly, I might add cynically, when queer politics is overshadowed by the "pink pound," or when, in the words of Valerie Lehr, "economic calculation replaces political debate as consumers replace citizens."[83] But if the bubble bursts, the doors may slam shut again; and then once again we may hear, as Yeats put it, "the ghost of Roger Casement . . . beating at the door."

2

Fetal Ireland
Reproduction, Agency, and Irish National Discourses

Unionists must ensure that nationalists don't outnumber them.
On the other side what are we confined to—outbreeding them?
What are our choices? Either we shoot them or we outbreed
them. There's no politics here. It's a numbers game.
—Bernadette Devlin McAliskey, Northern Irish activist

I think it's absolutely disgraceful that we, as Irish Republicans,
are discussing approval for the destruction of the future
members of the Irish nation.
—Máire Ward, Sinn Féin

Interpreting boundaries . . . is a way to contest them, not to
record their fixity in the natural world. Like penetrating Cuban
territory with reconnaissance satellites and Radio Marti,
treating a fetus as if it were outside a woman's body, because it
can be viewed, is a political act.
—Rosalind Pollack Petchesky, American feminist scholar

Borders matter. Critical theory has pushed borders, examined borders,
realigned them, transgressed them, exploded them. A border is a way to
imagine the limits of power, mobility, and the body in space. But borders, of course, are more than abstractions. National borders do exist
and, as is clear in Northern Ireland, are often contested and policed.

Another contested border is that which defines the limits of a
woman's body. Women's bodies, to use a now-hackneyed phrase, are

battlegrounds. The particular aptness of this metaphor is clear to anyone who has participated in or witnessed an abortion clinic defense/siege. Not only are the street, parking lot, and clinic the ground on which the battle is fought, but the bodies of the women who seek counseling and abortion are besieged, guarded by uniformed escorts, protected, and attacked. Perhaps somewhat more metaphorically, however, women's bodies are the site of ideological battle—a battle with far-reaching material consequences.

In order to explore the connections between the ideological and the material, I revisit the debates over the Irish constitutional amendment in the early 1980s, the infamous X Case of 1992 and concurrent Maastricht Treaty debates, the subsequent amendments to the Constitution, and the recent brief debates in the Northern Ireland Assembly over extending Great Britain's 1967 Abortion Act to Northern Ireland. Because the state relies on women for the perpetuation of its population, I argue in this chapter that there is a more than coincidental similarity between rhetorical constructions of the nation/state and the rhetorical construction of the fetus: both are fantasies of inviolability and autonomy, fantasies at odds with the much more complex ideological and material conditions of both entities. The similarity between fetus and nation/state points to the necessary but often discursively obscured link between the "private" choices of women and the "public" interests of the nation/state: the latter must control the former in order to reproduce itself. The nation/state's suppression of female agency is explored, and the distinction between private and public is exploded, in the works of a number of Irish artists whom I also consider in this chapter.

Conceiving the Nation: Fetal Ireland in the 1980s

The first wave of abortion debates in the Republic of Ireland reached their peak in the early 1980s, in the time leading up to the 1983 abortion referendum. At stake at the time was not only women's agency over their bodies, but also the permeability of the borders between the Republic of Ireland and the rest of Europe, as Laury Oaks has noted.[1] According to an article in *Magill,* the anti-abortion forces, represented by the Pro-Life Amendment Campaign (PLAC), were concerned with "the trends in sexual permissiveness, decline in ethical values and high abortion rates that have developed in other countries."[2] The PLAC groups were joined by a number of organizations, "mostly Catholic," who saw the abortion issue as "the last line of defense against the encroaching moral decadence of Europe"—a position that bears a striking similarity to reactions against homosexuality.[3] The anti-abortion amendment, it is worth pointing out, was to be legally redundant: the unchallenged 1861 Offenses Against the Person Act, Sections 58 and 59, makes intentional miscarriage a felony act liable to a life sentence of penal servitude and makes anyone assisting such an act guilty of a misdemeanor.[4] The amendment was thus intended not to criminalize abortion but to protect "life of the unborn," in the language of PLAC, from the threat of forces ostensibly outside of Ireland. Both pro-choice and queer politics suggested a threat to morality, morality defined primarily through the Catholic Church but also, given the extent to which Europe is here figured as the threat, defined as a particularly Irish kind of morality. As Oaks writes, "In Ireland, reproduction is a medium through which competing national origin stories that focus on Irish national identity and cultural self-determination, indeed visions of 'Irishness' itself, are imagined and expressed" ("Irishness," 133). Both the anti-abortion and the anti-homosexual positions imply a desire for the reproduction of a particular kind of Irishness, one that contains Irishness in the tightly circumscribed discourse of the heterosexual family cell.

"Reproduction" is a key term here, for what are, I would argue, more than metaphorical reasons. The concern over "encroaching moral decadence" in the 1980s masked a concern about Ireland's seeming inability to keep its population intact and within its borders. As Oaks notes, population loss during the 1845–48 potato blight and mass emigration in the 1980s and early 1990s fueled the fear that the Irish nation was in jeopardy, at risk of "dying out." Long influenced by the Catholic Church's strictures against contraception and abortion, however, the government prior to this time had not needed legislation to officially prevent abortion. The link between Catholicism and the national interest has ensured that the Catholic Church has a central role in the Irish State, despite the 1972 repeal of Article 44, section 2, of the 1937 Irish Constitution in which "The State recognizes the special position of the Holy Catholic Apostolic and Roman Church as the guardian of the Faith professed by the great majority of its citizens."[5]

The relationship between reproduction and the national interest is also reflected in an earlier section of the Constitution: *Bunreacht na hÉireann* officially insists that women's place is in the home and that women bear the responsibility of the family. Although this fact has been much commented upon, it bears repeating. Under the section of "Fundamental Rights" entitled "The Family" (Article 41), the Constitution states the following:

> 1. 1° The State recognizes the Family as the natural primary and fundamental unit group of Society, and as a moral institution possessing inalienable and imprescriptible rights, antecedent and superior to all positive law.
>
> 2° The State, therefore, guarantees to protect the Family in its constitution and authority, as the necessary basis of social order and as indispensable to the welfare of the Nation and the State.
>
> 2. 1° In particular, the State recognizes that by her life within the home, woman gives to the State a support without which the common good cannot be achieved.
>
> 2° The State shall, therefore, endeavour to ensure that mothers shall not be obliged by economic necessity to engage in labour to the neglect of their duties in the home.[6]

Ruth Riddick has pointed out that "woman" and "mother" are seen as interchangeable terms in the Irish Constitution, as can be seen from the rhetorical move from 2.1 to 2.2: it is clear that mothers are the only women the state deems worth acknowledging.[7] In the Irish context, the combination of the pro-natalist Catholic Church and the domestic patriarchy insisted on by the Constitution combine to ensure that the concerns of reproducing the Irish national subject and maintaining the family cell rest firmly on the shoulders of Irish women.

The debates about abortion in Ireland have thus never focused on population control, despite the nation/state's interest in reproducing itself. Instead, the nationalist concern has been framed in terms of the morality—or, more to the point, the immorality—of the individual reproductive choices of Irish women. Framing reproduction in terms of "choice," as American feminist legal scholar Catharine MacKinnon has suggested, assumes that women have agency within the private sphere; but "privacy is by no means a gender-neutral concept," as one can see in, for instance, the Irish Constitution. "The existing distribution of power and resources within the private sphere," MacKinnon asserts, "[is] what the law of privacy exists to protect."[8] The reproductive "choices" with which Irish women are faced impact more than the private sphere: they are the basis of the reproduction of the nation/state. As Lauren Berlant has suggested in her discussion of American fetal-rights and citizenship discourse, "The reproducing woman is no longer cast as a potentially productive citizen, except insofar as she procreates: her capacity for other kinds of creative agency has become an obstacle for national reproduction."[9] Women's agency, in other words, must be curtailed and put to the service of the family cell if the nation/state is to reproduce itself. It is in the nation/state's interest to support those discourses that assist in its own reproduction; and anti-abortion discourse provides such assistance in its idealization of the fetus and its demonization of female agency over reproduction.

Medical technologies have at the very least assisted, if not actually created, the discursive construction of the autonomous fetus. As Rosalind Pollack Petchesky has argued, fetal imaging techniques take the fetus out of the context of the womb and the woman, thus representing the fetus as a discrete and independent subject. Petchesky notes that "fetal imagery epitomizes the distortion inherent in all photographic images: the tendency to slice up reality into tiny bits wrenched out of real space and time, which leads to seeing reality as data "divorced from historical process or social relationships."[10] The fetus is taken out of the context of the narrative of the pregnant woman of which it is inextricably a part and is renarrativized as a separate autonomous subject — as evidenced, for instance, by the "pro-life" film *The Silent Scream* in which fetal development in the womb is recontextualized, without the apparently irrelevant pregnant woman, as a kind of life story. *The Silent Scream* emerges out of the history of the popular use of fetal imaging that can be traced, as Petchesky notes, back at least as far as an article in *Look* magazine publicizing a book entitled *The First Nine Months of Life*, in which the fetus is constantly pictured as a solitary entity and is referred to as "the baby" (268), and which includes such representations as the Star Child of *2001: A Space Odyssey*, an autonomous being floating in empty space.[11] Fetal technology has meant that the pregnant woman is reduced to "the maternal environment" (277), a kind of passive landscape of fetal growth and "life."

The Society for the Protection of Unborn Children (SPUC), an initially London-based anti-choice group, relied and continues to rely upon this imagery in its pamphlets. In one pamphlet, "Threatened by a Human Rights Body," it goes so far as to picture "a baby only six weeks after conception" in an amniotic sac, dangling from male hands, in order to impress upon viewers the human development of the embryo. The image reinforces the notion that the fetus is an autonomous entity; as it dangles there in its entirety, no comment is made about why it has been removed from the mother's womb and whether it was a viable fetus. The text comments that "at about twenty-four days after conception the baby's heart begins to beat and will continue until the end of his or her life," avoiding the fact that the fetus that illustrates this narrative cannot be "the baby" whose heart the text describes as beating.[12]

The threat the pamphlet constructs, however, comes not from the male hands that dangle "the baby": it implicitly comes from the "maternal landscape," typically constructed by anti-abortion discourse as a hostile one. Ruth Riddick points out that "during the [Irish anti-abortion] amendment campaign, and subsequently, it was claimed that the womb . . . was no less than 'the most dangerous place in the world to be'—this in a world with the nuclear capacity to annihilate all life many times over."[13] Berlant notes the tendency in American anti-abortion discourse to construct the fetus in the language of the marginalized: "The pro-life movement has composed a magical and horrifying spectacle of amazing vulnerability: the unprotected person, the citizen without a country or future, the fetus unjustly imprisoned in its mother's hostile gulag" (150). The SPUC pamphlet described above works on this assumption, asking its audience to "VALUE YOUR VOICE—VALUE YOUR VOTE. Make it count for those with no voice and no vote." The "you" is, of course, not the pregnant woman; the audience is exhorted to speak for the imprisoned fetus in a clear mimicking of civil rights discourse employed by politically disenfranchised and marginalized peoples. Women's agency is either erased or seen as threatening; in the Irish context, women are either the landscape for Ireland's "unborn citizens" or the primary enemy of the fetus, depending on which argument the anti-abortion rhetoric is being used to advance. In either case the anti-abortion forces stand opposed to women's agency.

The anti-abortion activists' rhetorical spin on the issue of ectopic pregnancy and uterine cancer during the amendment campaign is a clear example of the ways in which anti-abortion discourse attempted to contain pregnant women's agency. Dr. Julia Vaughan of PLAC wrote to the *Irish Times* that the removal of a fetus in such circumstances was not abortion: "In each case the removal of a pathological organ is carried out to save the woman's life, not in order to kill the foetus. The pregnancy is not directly attacked, even though its loss may be an inevitable consequence of treatment which has as its primary objective the 'good' of saving the mother's life."[14] Her language suggests that what is of primary importance is the *intent* of the action, performed for the woman by a physician, even though the outcome is the same whether or not the pregnant woman actively sought the removal of her fetus. This rhetorical tendency to remove the pregnant woman's agency from the pregnancy

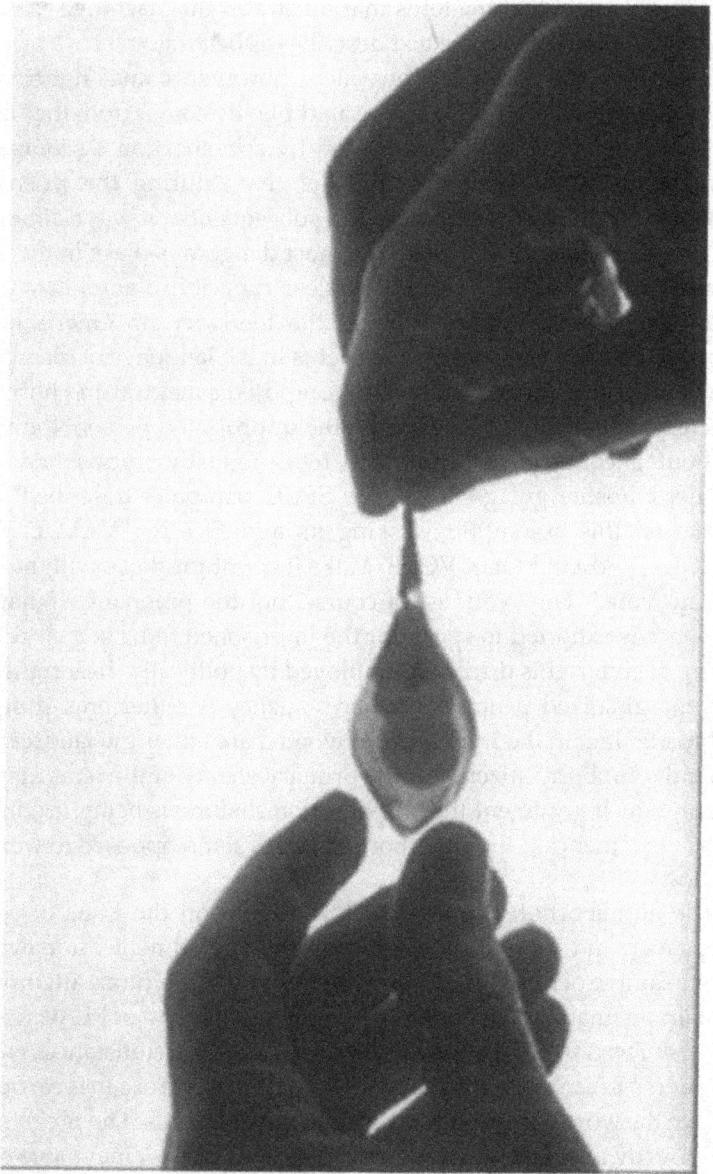

Fetal image from Society for the Protection of Unborn Children
pamphlet, ca. 1990s

continued throughout the pro-amendment campaign. Dr. Mary Lucey of SPUC wrote to the *Irish Times* on September 20, 1982: "Every new life is a miracle of the Lord of creation. . . . There is a new human person whose heart is beating even before the mother knows she is pregnant. To those who say there is nothing only a blob of jelly or a piece of jelly from the first moment: there is a separate human being living within the womb, dependent on the mother but not a part of her. This can all be medically demonstrated and proven. That being true, is it not obvious that the unborn person has a right to life?" (quoted in Hesketh, 48). Lucey's language emphasizes that God, not the pregnant woman, brings forth life—a key point in much Catholic pro-amendment discourse. But more important, Lucey creates distance between pregnant woman and fetus. She argues that the heart of the "unborn person" beats "even before the mother knows she is pregnant," suggesting that the pregnant woman is alienated from her own body. She also states that the fetus is not "part of" the mother, further distancing the autonomous "unborn person" from the pregnant woman via the "authority" of medicine. Lucey's letter exemplifies the rhetorical violence done to the pregnant woman under the rubric of medical "knowledge" about the fetus, here combined for double effect with religious authority.

In short, epistemology is political, as suggested by the Petchesky epigraph that begins this chapter. She compares the penetration of the womb by imaging techniques to the penetration of Cuban space by American anti-Castro radio programming. The parallel between the two cases seems to be that neither radio signals nor imaging techniques are politically neutral. Petchesky recognizes that borders are being manipulated and contested in both cases. Her statement, however, implies that one *should* "record [the fixity of borders] in the natural world," though to do so means accepting the problematic "natural," the same terminology that consigns women to the "natural" role of mother. Squier suggests seeing "fetal/maternal relations as a border, a creative space of contestation, both linguistic and experimental." Though Squier does wish to resist the "tendencies to split the fetus from the gestating woman," imagining the fetal-maternal relationship as a border already defines the two beings as in conflict, further reinforcing the discursive construction of the autonomous fetus at odds with either the colonizing pregnant woman or the threatening "maternal environment."[15] Squier cites Barbara Katz Rothman, who provides a somewhat more workable rhetorical model in which "women and their fetuses are bound together, and enmeshed in a social world."[16] Such a model acknowledges the inseparability of the gestation narrative of the fetus (the "first nine months of life") from that of the narrative of a woman's pregnancy and life.

Such a rhetorical model is dangerous to the stable reproduction of the nation, however. Women's bodies, Berlant notes, are useful only insofar as they reproduce stable identities; the pregnant woman becomes "an identity machine for others" (147). But a woman with agency over her fetus has control over the "potential citizen," and given the logic of the fetus-as-individual, the pregnant woman also threatens to become a double subject, I would argue. She can speak both for herself *and* with and for the fetus—the latter a position currently assumed by doctors, celebrities, and politicians, as Berlant notes and the Irish anti-abortion discourse emphasizes. The corporeal contingency of pregnant woman and fetus—the fluidity of the boundary between them—potentially gives women double weight; the mother who "speaks for two" challenges the fixity of boundaries and identities. Such a challenge threatens not only anti-abortion discourse but also a national discourse that depends on women's silence, passivity, and acceptance of their place in the family cell to ensure its perpetuation.

The fetus alone, however, is pure potential citizen, a sign of the reproduction of the nation/state.[17] But even further, I would suggest that there is a synecdochic similarity between the fetus's relationship to the mother and Ireland's relationship to Europe. The fantasy of the fetus as an uncorrupted and autonomous entity in Irish nationalist, anti-abortion discourse is also a fantasy of the security and autonomy of Ireland. As goes the fetus, so goes the nation; all the hopes of the latter are pinned on the purity and security of the former entity. But this construction also exposes fears about the vulnerability of both the fetus and the nation/state. Feminist scholar Ailbhe Smyth has commented on the ways in which Ireland has been figured in "extreme-right ideology and politics" as under threat:

> An important strand in extreme-right ideology and politics in Ireland since the 1970s has been the emphasis on Ireland as the last bastion of moral and sexual purity and of the traditional family in the Western world. In this scenario, Ireland plays the heroic role of the tiny beleaguered State staunchly defending the Faith of Our Fathers (and the invisibility of our mothers) by holding out against the global wave of depravity which threatens to engulf it, and thus (somewhat illogically) Ireland shines as a beacon for all those in need of salvation. . . . Those—especially women—who go the way of all flesh and "choose" divorce, contraception, or abortion are therefore traitors to both Church and State.

The message is that Ireland must and *can* save the world from dissolution and destruction. This would be merely ludicrous if it did not so wittingly appeal to a need for status and self-importance in the collective Irish psyche. For whatever Irish people may like to think, the fact is that Ireland is an insignificant geographical, economic, and political entity in the European and, *a fortiori*, global scheme of things.[18]

Smyth's comments suggest that Ireland's needs for "self-aggrandizement" come from its status as "an ex-colonial state, with an insecure sense of national identity," one that finds itself in an uncertain relationship with a strengthening Europe. She notes that its need for a raison d'être in this context is "understandable but disturbing when one of the chief ways, de facto, it has achieved a distinctive identity within Europe is through its denial to women of full citizenship rights" (120). The notion of a fetus contiguous with a woman who is an agent over her own body, I would argue, parallels the position of Ireland in this strengthening Europe, inseparably linked with European cultures and economies. But this notion challenges the vision of the autonomous Irish fetus as Irish citizen, the pure and unsullied hope for future Irish potential, "uncorrupted" by adult politics (such as economics, reproductive rights, and political agency). Accepting the pregnant woman as agent means acknowledging simultaneously that the narratives both of fetus and mother *and* of the Irish nation and the rest of the world are linked. In order to ensure the uncomplicated perpetuation of the Irish nation-state, then, women's agency over their bodies must be contained both by perpetuating the heterosexual family cell and by limiting women's access to reproductive choices: the narrative of women's lives and the future of the nation-state are inextricably linked.

"Something Big": Responses to the Death of Ann Lovett

The year 1983 saw the passage of the Eighth Amendment to the Irish Constitution, following the long and intense campaign on behalf of the "fetal citizen." Article 40 ("Personal Rights"), section 3.3, states, "The State acknowledges the right to life of the unborn and, with due regard to the equal right to life of the mother, guarantees in its laws to respect, and as far as practicable, by its laws to defend and vindicate that right."[19] The amendment passed by 66.45 percent (Riddick, 143). The debate was, however, far from over: the abortion debates were linked with a number of controversial cases, including the death of Sheila Hodgers, who died without painkillers of a cancer that doctors did not treat because she was pregnant; fifteen-year-old Ann Lovett's death in childbirth alone at the grotto of the Virgin Mary at Granard; and the infamous Kerry Babies Case. All the cases concerned the tension between the private and the public and the silencing of women's voices in the discussion of women's agency over their bodies.

The death of Ann Lovett in particular inspired an outpouring of creative responses from Irish writers. Elizabeth Butler Cullingford cites Nuala ní Dhomhnaill's poem "*Thar mo Chionn*," Sinéad O'Connor's and Christy Moore's song "Middle of the Island," Leland Bardwell's short story "The Dove of Peace," and Paula Meehan's poem "The Statue of the Virgin at Granard Speaks" as works conceived in response to that tragedy, all of which point to the troubling relationships between church, state, the family cell, and individual women.[20]

Published three years after the death of Ann Lovett but set in the early years of the Republic, Bardwell's "The Dove of Peace" articulates a powerful criticism of the silence that surrounds the Irish family and the abuse that can result from the maintenance of "privacy" at the expense of female children's lives. The text is framed by a first-person narration by an older woman who begins by noting "there's a hole in my memory."[21] Her knowledge of her memory loss is juxtaposed with her pastime, the making of boxes—an activity that represents a perhaps subconscious effort at the containment of a painful past. The boxes are more explicitly tied to that containment when she notes that she has "made boxes inlaid with garnets and coloured glass set in garlands of flowers resembling the wild herbaceous borders of the big house where she and I used to play" (7). This is the first mention of another person, and to whom "she" refers remains unclear until after we learn that the death of the narrator's father in 1946, many years prior to the textual present, has "given me back my past": for four years, she had lost most of her memory of her childhood. Just before the narrative shifts to third person, the narrator names the other "she": "Columbine, my Dove of Peace," the narrator's older sister (9).

The main story is one of incest between Columbine and her father. The narrator of the frame and, by inference, the incest story is Jessica, whose name we learn as the narrative switches from first to third person. That switch is one of several markers of Jessica's/the narrator's attempt to distance herself from the traumatic events of the core story and to box those events in. Another is her attempt, as a child, to rationalize the "nightly terrors" she experiences: "It was only at night that a strange anomaly manifested itself. Jessica never quite knew when she found out the cause of her nightly terrors. It was like a gradual growth of the faculties, the inculcation of logic into her childish brain. These nocturnal noises had, after all, a human origin. There were no ghosts, no disembodied spirits, nothing, in fact, to be afraid of. It was only Daddy, who came up to give Columbine a last goodnight kiss, to hold her soft body in his arms, reassure her of his love" (10–11). The "logic" Jessica is pressured to learn is the logic of the family and of privacy: since there is no supernatural threat from without, there is no threat. According to this "logic," the inviolate personal space of the family cell ensures — or is believed to ensure — safety.

The "logic" with which she has been imbued, however, is followed immediately by the beginning of her lifelong pastime, making boxes — another attempt to distance herself from the incest happening in her presence. She teaches herself how to build them, using cast-off pieces of furniture and an abandoned bag of tools in a shed at the end of the garden. She becomes "obsessed," her pastime a "secret obsession": "no one must know about her boxes. Especially Columbine" (11). The boxes allow her to create another "secret," private space that she believes to be safe from others. The boxes can be read as a metaphor for a female sexuality over which Jessica has control: she is able to choose what goes in and out of those containers. But the boxes are also a metaphor for silence and containment, which ironically help to ensure and protect from outside intervention the very "nightly terrors" that Jessica attempts to shut out with her obsession.

Jessica's persistent but "logical" naiveté leads her to misread the cause of her mother's psychological distress, which manifests itself as, alternately, wandering and staring. Jessica's naiveté, however, does create an interesting metaphoric tension between the incest and her creation of boxes. The following exchange takes place between Jessica and Columbine:

> "What is wrong with Mammy?" Jessica asked.
> "She's mad. Stone mad."
> "Why is she mad?"
> "She's mad because she can't have what she wants."
> "What does she want?"
> "Something big, Daddy says."
> "What does that mean?"
> "Dunno." (11–12)

Jessica assumes that her mother literally needs any large object in order to be satisfied; unsatisfied with the size of her boxes, she buys a toy elephant, which, she hopes, will stand in for "something big." When she offers the gift along with her father's statement as explanation, however, her mother strikes her repeatedly and eventually is picked up by a white van to go to a "mad house" (13). Jessica's original impulse to make a box is, in a roundabout way, in keeping with the original intent of the father's statement. The father presumably intends "something big" to mean his penis, but both the boxes Jessica makes and the father's penis are symbols of privacy, the privileges of which are denied to Jessica's mother. The boxes work both literally and metaphorically to distract attention away from the incest, to contain it within the private sphere, the space of male privilege.

Once the mother leaves the house, the sisters adopt the role of homemaker without question. The evening visits to Columbine continue, although one night her father leaves seemingly inexplicably. Columbine informs Jessica that she has "her visitor": Jessica assumes that this "visitor" is somehow connected to the visitations of her father at night. Of course, the "visitor" is Columbine's period, but once again Jessica's naiveté is logical: both the father's visitations and Columbine's menstruation are handled with silence and distance, part of the sexuality that is simultaneously denied and forced upon them. Like unwelcome visitors, menstruation and incest are inconveniences accepted silently, following an unwritten code of propriety.

This code of silence is reinforced by the townspeople once Columbine discovers that she is pregnant. The headmistress of the school insists on disclosure but combines her disapproval of the baby's father with the assumption of Columbine's guilt: "'Who is the father? You must tell me. So he can be punished too. God has punished you for your sin and will go on punishing you all the days of your life'" (18). Neither Columbine nor Jessica disclose that their father is "the father": the headmistress's accusation serves further to reinforce the myth of Columbine's agency in the incest and suggests the collaboration of paternal and religious authority in that myth. When Jessica encourages Columbine to vent her rage at her father, the latter answers, "'It's my fault, Jessica. He couldn't help it'" (19). The girls internalize this myth of agency, enforced by such seemingly innocuous comments as "Columbine can charm the birds off the trees" (9); this internalization guarantees their silence.

As the story draws to a close, Jessica notes the absence of her sister and recognizes with panic that she has probably gone to give birth. She first assumes that Columbine is in the shed, that site of silent, distracted box making. She realizes that Columbine is not there, and the narration shifts abruptly and unexpectedly back to the first person as Jessica finishes the tale of her search for her sister. Her shouts rouse the neighbors who, she now realizes, were all along "exulting in my sister's pregnancy" (22). Jessica escapes from them after they try to silence her with pills and eventually finds her sister lying still in a ditch beyond a neighboring farm, with a dead child at her feet.

Near the end of the story, the narrator alludes again to the "hole in her memory" with which the story began—but it is not wholly clear what she has forgotten other than the moments after the discovery of her sister. Jessica asks, "Did I die then with her . . . ?" (23), a continuation, perhaps, of her mimicking of her sister Columbine's behavior and, later, her pregnancy: "Jessica felt that she was pregnant, too, that she was also shielding the child from prying eyes. She began to walk as Columbine, take on her habits, just as she had as a small child" (20). Jessica's mirroring of her sister's behavior, while typical of siblings, suggests the possibility that the existence of her sister is yet another form of distancing created by the narrator: like the boxes (which, we discover at the end, have made her rich and famous) and the third-person narration, Columbine is perhaps another creative response to abuse and incest, a "dove of peace" who carries the pain of Jessica's own experience of abuse away from her. Each narrative possibility reproduces another silencing, another "box" out of which it becomes difficult to extract the "truth" of incest; each "memory failure" ensures that the narrative will be reproduced only in part, contained by the "logic" of patriarchal privilege.

Whether Columbine is meant to exist literally or is merely another facet of the narrator's experience, however, the story "The Dove of Peace" breaks open the narrative box of silence by articulating the unspeakable about incest and the way it is fostered by "privacy." And the narrator's memory loss is a metaphor for the repetition of the narrative of silence and abuse across the years: "I feel the failing memory of the old . . . the difficulty in distinguishing one decade from another" (7). Though the narrator decides at one point to "let sleeping dogs lie," the narrative itself exceeds the box in which she has put it, breaking abruptly at the end from third to first person, from distanced object to subject. Nonetheless, her confusion about her memories bespeaks the ease with which the injunction to be quiet, not to interfere, is internalized by those whom silence does not protect. When read against the story of Ann Lovett, "The Dove of Peace" presents the obvious outcome of continued silence: the death of young women.

Ann Lovett's death resonates through many of the artistic responses to the abortion amendment, serving as a focal point for the desire to address the mechanisms that continued to foster silence at the expense both of women's agency and women's lives. Paula Meehan's poem "The Statue of the Virgin at Granard Speaks," published several years after the death of Ann Lovett, explores the repression of women at the hands of an institutional authority structure—in this case, the Catholic Church. The Virgin statue-as-Mary, the narrative persona of the poem, recounts the way she has been idealized by the Church:

> They call me Mary—Blessed, Holy, Virgin.
> They fit me to the myth of a man crucified:
> the scourging and the falling, and the falling again,
> the thorny crown, the hammer blow of iron
> into wrist and ankle, the sacred bleeding heart.
> They name me Mother of all this grief
> though mated to no mortal man.
>
> (ll. 20–26)

These lines suggest the way in which Mary's identity has been sub-sumed into the "larger" narrative of Christ's death. They also suggest the negative side to idealization: though she is the mother of Christ, she is also the mother of grief, responsible for the incarnation and thus the later material suffering of Christ on earth but yet not allowed the mate-rial pleasure of sexuality. Her desire to be like a live, human woman is emphasized as the poem progresses: "My being / cries out to be incar-nate, incarnate, / maculate and tousled in a honeyed bed" (ll. 40–42). Mary-as-statue cannot, however, realize her desires: she is trapped, both literally and figuratively, as an immaculate idealized image, incapable of any agency.

As with Jessica of "The Dove of Peace," Mary is haunted by her own immobility when she remembers the death of the fifteen-year-old girl:

> On a night like this I remember the child
> who came with fifteen summers to her name,
> and she lay down along at my feet
> without midwife or doctor or friend to hold her hand
> and she pushed her secret out into the night,
> far from the town tucked up in little scandals,
> bargains struck, words broken, prayers, promises,
> and though she cried out to me in extremis
> I did not move,
> I didn't lift a finger to help her,
> I didn't intercede with heaven,
> nor whisper the charmed word in God's ear.
>
> (ll. 56–67)

Mary's view of her own agency here suggests her internalization of the blame for the girl's death; though she is a statue who cannot, literally, "lift a finger," she nonetheless implies her own guilt by saying that she "did not" rather than "could not" help.

Her self-blame can also be read, at least in part, as the result of being the representative of a Church that has denied its responsibility for those who share the fate of the pregnant child, a Church that shares the secrets and broken promises of the town from which the girl came. Mary does, however, gesture outside the Church when she prays to the sun, "molten mother of us all," in the final stanza, asking that she "hear me and have pity" (ll. 73–74). This final prayer is an appeal for pity on Mary, to some degree, but more directly on those who have, with good or bad intentions ("men hunt each other and invoke / the various names of God as blessing / on their death tactics, their night manoeuvres"; ll. 13–15), placed their faith in an idealized image of the Church.

By making clear the inefficacy of the Church that the Virgin statue represents, Meehan's lamenting Mary exposes the system that locks her, and the women who appeal to her, into a position of no agency. And in so doing, Meehan, like Bardwell, makes the connection between ideological constructions of femininity and the material suffering than can result from them.

Women to Blame: The Kerry Babies Case

The silence about Ann Lovett's pregnancy and death revealed the collaboration of community, church, and institutional authority to keep the myth of the normative "healthy" patriarchal family cell intact. This coalition of forces reappeared later in April 1984, when a dead baby boy washed up onto the White Strand three miles from the town of Cahirciveen in County Kerry. The ensuing Kerry Babies Case not only reinforced the gendering of the privilege of privacy but also demonstrated the state's fear of women's agency and suggested the close relationship between the territory of women's bodies and national territories. After the baby was brought in, the state's pathologist pronounced the baby murdered, and the guards (the *gardaí*, or Irish police) immediately began to search for parents of the child. The search included canvassing the neighborhoods and questioning doctors and clergy in the area. With the help of a breach of confidentiality by a doctor, the guards decided that a twenty-four-year-old woman named Joanne Hayes might have given birth to the Cahirciveen baby. She had been pregnant, but there was no baby officially registered. The guards gathered confessions from each member of the family that suggested that Joanne had given birth to her child and then stabbed the baby to death; her siblings then drove the corpse to Slea Head and threw the baby into the sea. But as the confessions were being taken from the family, Joanne told her sister Kathleen where to find her baby, to which she had silently given stillbirth, on the family farm. The baby was found.

The Kerry Babies Case was thus intended to be a tribunal of inquiry into police conduct in the case—given the startling existence of several somewhat contradictory statements from a woman and her family "confessing" to being part of the murder of a baby to whom the woman in question could not have given birth. The inquiry was anything but an inquiry into police conduct, however. Instead, the investigation turned again toward Joanne Hayes: although charges against her had been dropped, the tribunal, consisting entirely of men, asked whether Joanne Hayes was perhaps so "loose" in her morals that she could have been impregnated by more than one man and thus have been pregnant with two fetuses and have given birth, on different days, to two children with two different fathers.

Journalist Nell McCafferty recounts the events leading up to and including the tribunal in *A Woman to Blame: The Kerry Babies Case*. McCafferty's text displays an awareness of the ways in which discourse can be formulated and wielded by the state to secure heteronormative "family values" and erase, or attempt to erase, indictments of the nation/state's ideological hegemony. McCafferty's text serves as an intervention into this hegemonic process by providing a counternarrative, one that explodes the distinction between the "public" and the "private."

Her prologue begins with an example of the extent to which privacy is a particularly male privilege:

> In the opening days of the "Kerry babies" tribunal a married man went to bed in a Tralee hotel with a woman who was not his wife. He was one of the forty-three male officials—judge, fifteen lawyers, three police superintendents and twenty-four policemen—engaged in a public probe of the private life of Joanne Hayes.
>
> When this particular married man was privately confronted with his own behaviour he at first denied it. Then he crumpled into tears and asked not to be exposed. He had so much to lose, he said. "My wife . . . my job . . . my reputation . . ." He was assured of discretion.
>
> No such discretion was assured to Joanne Hayes, as a succes-

sion of professional men, including this married man, came forward to strip her character. (7)

McCafferty foregrounds the issue of privacy and publicity, demonstrating the extent to which privacy works to maintain both male privilege and the fantasy of the coherent family cell, reinforcing MacKinnon's point that "women have no privacy to lose or guarantee" (MacKinnon, 191). Once the Cahirciveen baby had been found by the police, the private became public in the search for the killer of the baby. The details of the case were spread conversationally by the police chief, Donal Sullivan, in order, in his own words, "to get the rumour around and get the word on the streets." Those who did not fit the profile of members of the normative family cell were investigated for the murder: "hippies," "travelling families," "a man with a criminal record and a common-law wife," "a pregnant woman known to have paid a visit to England." She notes that "the police were even given the name of a woman who had been prescribed certain tablets to help in her pregnancy. The name of the informant was confidential, of course." McCafferty writes that "one woman did benefit from the unexpected intrusion into her private life." She had given secret birth to a child; the guards came, registered the child, and a welfare officer encouraged her to register for the unmarried mother's benefit of fifty-one pounds a week. McCafferty notes with some irony that "[the woman] and her mother, with the child in the pram, are still to be seen daily scavenging the town dump. A financial safety net of some kind has been provided" (11–12).

The Irish Constitution does not explicitly guarantee the right to privacy, but privacy has been legally constructed as a right, and "the private" is invoked strategically by the state in order to protect the primacy of the heterosexual family cell.[22] The privacy afforded the adulterous officer of the tribunal was not afforded Joanne Hayes or the "hippies" in Kerry precisely because to do so would be to allow the alternative forms of "family" represented by those people to exist unchallenged. The death of the Cahirciveen baby posed a problem to a state that had just passed an anti-abortion amendment and had insisted that "the most dangerous place to be at the moment is in the mother's womb"; it was only seven months later that they were to find "a baby that had safely escaped the womb, only to meet instant death" (McCafferty, 10). The investigation of Joanne Hayes thus refocused attention on the criminal deviance of this specific and ostensibly abnormal woman and her family—declared by the tribunal judge, Kevin Lynch, to be "very odd"

(83)—rather than the more generalized problem of the limits on women's reproductive freedom that produced, among other things, the high instance of infanticide in Ireland. The official sleight-of-hand is similarly demonstrated, McCafferty notes, in the rhetorical construction of the death of Ann Lovett at Granard, and the subsequent suicide of her fourteen-year-old sister, as "a private family tragedy" (10). The "private" is here invoked to maintain the illusion of functionality of the "moral institution" of the family on which the perpetuation of the Irish nation/state ostensibly depends: to investigate these deaths would mean exposing the family, "indispensable to the welfare of the Nation and the State" (*Bunreacht*, 136), to critical reevaluation.

McCafferty's text reclaims the public sphere by naming, whenever possible, those involved in the proceedings. The "discretion" of privacy afforded to men in this case is resisted whenever possible. She also explodes the distinction between the "private" sphere, ostensibly beyond the arm of the state, and officially confidential proceedings, suggesting the extent to which the myth of free choice is maintained in both settings through official state ignorance. The most obvious example of the state's abuse of privacy or secrecy is the setting in which the confessions were extracted, described in the chapter appropriately entitled "Behind Closed Doors." Once Joanne Hayes's baby was found and the charges were dropped, the family explained to an internal police inquiry the intimidation tactics employed by the police to get the family to confirm the police's accusations. The police responded that the family's "presence in the police station was purely voluntary and they were free to leave any time they wished" (73). McCafferty points to the ways in which the state masks its own agency in the manipulation of the private sphere; the myth that the state hoped to maintain was both that the family had free choice and that the state would have no investment in limiting that choice. After the police pressure tactics failed, McCafferty notes with some sarcasm, "the inquiry aborted" (74). By ironically constructing the end of the inquiry as a passive, spontaneous "abortion," McCafferty suggests that the state's investment in the anti-abortion campaign had much in common with the inquiry into the allegations of police misconduct. In both cases, the state deflected attention away from its own actions and toward the negative outcome of what appeared to be free choices made by individual citizens.

The state's choice to focus attention on the morally suspect Joanne Hayes and her family led the police to concoct or coerce from the family

certain narratives that supposedly explained the death of the Cahirciveen baby. McCafferty reproduces the confessions in full in her text. She
notes, too, the odd discrepancies and contradictions in their statements.
"Had there been perfect accord between the statements," argued the
police chief, "it would have looked suspicious" (68). These narratives
helped to create the identity of Joanne Hayes-as-murderer, defined
wholly in terms of her purported actions on the night of the birth and
death of the Cahirciveen baby. Later, as the tribunal investigating the
guards progressed, Joanne Hayes's "identity" was fleshed out through
selective additions to the narrative leading up to the birth of her child —
or children, as the investigators still suggested. The repetition of certain
details of her life — her sexual activity with a married man; her status as
a single mother who, according to one psychiatrist, had "got herself
pregnant on three occasions" (163); and eventually the insistence, based
on her demeanor in court, on her so-called "histrionic personality"
(161) — all helped to naturalize the narrative that supported the claim to
superfecundation, or the simultaneous existence of two fetuses by two
different fathers to which she might have given birth on two different
days. This narrative of Joanne Hayes's life, manipulated by the tribunal
with very little input from Hayes herself, became so fixed in the minds
of those on the tribunal that the scientific evidence supporting her innocence became irrelevant to them. Even though the superfecundation
theory was challenged and eventually ruled out, "'there were times
when we all thought she had twins,' said judge Kevin Lynch" (169).

　McCafferty's text, however, serves to disrupt the repetition of narratives designed to invent and naturalize the idea of Joanne Hayes as a
murderer: while she presents those narratives, she simultaneously
places Hayes in the larger discourse surrounding women's agency in
Ireland. She names the players who had publicly supported the pro-life
amendment (38); she discusses the attitudes of local doctors and phar-
macists who felt it was their duty to decide who were appropriate re-
cipients of contraception (30–33); she recounts the events that occurred
before and during the Kerry Babies Case, such as the death of Sheila
Hodgers (38), the death of Ann Lovett (10), and the anti-abortion campaign (10, 37–39). She notes also that "[Taoiseach/Prime Minister] Charlie Haughey, who was against contraception for single people then and
now, and against abortion for anyone, came to Kerry during the
[amendment] campaign to commemorate the life and death of a party
member who had fought with the IRA in the 1916 rising. . . . The man of

whom he spoke used to kill people" (38). For anyone who thinks that anti-abortion discourse in Ireland centers primarily on the moral belief that abortion is murder, Haughey's celebration of the IRA member might seem ironic. But as I have suggested above, Irish anti-abortion discourse is in part an arm of the nation-state, concerned with reproducing itself. In that light, Haughey's behavior is perfectly consistent. McCafferty also describes the community in which the events took place, Abbeydorney, a small parish in Kerry. Throughout the 1930s, Abbeydorney was at the mercy of Eamon DeValera's economic war with England. The community, however, rallied around the Catholic Young Men's Society, which demonized trade unions as "red infiltration" and bolstered a xenophobic Irish nationalism (17). At the same time, a Public Dance Halls Act was passed that prevented people from more than three miles away from entering a dance hall; the act was intended to "preserve the morals of the local community" (18). Though seemingly unconnected to the Kerry Babies Case, all these details place the case in the larger context of an Irish national discourse that contains and limits acceptable behaviors in the interests of maintaining the state. And McCafferty similarly places Joanne Hayes in the context of this larger narrative, highlighting not only the extent to which Hayes's behavior and choices were circumscribed by the discourse that surrounded her, but also the perfect logic of the way in which her case was handled. By renarrativizing the events, McCafferty suggests the larger discourse of which Hayes was a part, answering, to some degree, the question asked by the judge, with which she ends the book: "'What have the women of Ireland got to do with this case?'" (169).

The tremendous outpouring of support by women across the country that McCafferty records also answers the judge's question: women across the country saw in Joanne Hayes a potential image of themselves. Kate Shanahan, a Dublin activist involved in a group called Women for Disarmament, commented that the experience of seeing Joanne Hayes and her mother made her and other women realize "how close we all are to disaster if the public should be given a look in at us" (130). Her statement suggests that women are not necessarily part of "the public," that the "public interest" is not the same as a woman's interests. Her comment speaks volumes about the lack of women's "place": not protected by privacy, not acknowledged as part of the public sphere, women are the landscape on which the nation-state's interests are written.

Part(ur)ition: The Amendment, the North, and the Politics of Containment

That landscape—the landscape of Ireland and of Irish women—remained a site of contestation throughout the 1980s, and the two were linked in fairly concrete ways. The 1983 abortion referendum symbolically fixed even more solidly the border between North and South. Before the election, several politicians, religious leaders, and others, North and South, opposed the amendment on the grounds that it would serve to reinforce the Northern Unionist assumption that the South was a Catholic state. The issue was one of states' political boundaries, not women's political agency. In the South, Capuchin Father Brendan O'Mahony expressed early opposition to the amendment on the grounds that to "impose the view of the majority religion" was "moral and religious imperialism" (quoted in Hesketh, 64–65). The editor of the *Irish Times,* on July 3, 1982, wrote that the amendment "should be dropped forever . . . for, whatever the motives of the originators, it is not only inappropriate among all the gush we have had about ecumenism, but is inimical to the interests of a united Ireland" (quoted in Hesketh, 101). The Irish Council of Trade Unions (ICTU) backed the Anti-Amendment Campaign (AAC) and Tom Bogue, president of the Local Government and Public Services Union and staff officer with the Cork County Council, expressed concern that the amendment would "reinforce the views of those who believed that the Republic was a Catholic state" (Hesketh 93). But perhaps most surprising was a memo on Haughey's proposed amendment from the Department of Foreign Affairs, dated September 20, 1982, and written on behalf of the minister: "Given the Government's commitment to fostering reconciliation between the two major traditions in Ireland, it is necessary to examine carefully any proposal which attracts the unanimous condemnation of Unionist politicians who will see in it the introduction of a sectarian provision into the Constitution and confirmation thereby of the view that the State is a Roman Catholic State which aspires to Irish Unity, so as to impose domination on the Protestant people of Northern Ireland. Reservations have accordingly been expressed about the proposal by Roman Catholics in Northern Ireland (including Senator Seamus Mallon)" (quoted in Hesketh, 151–52). The AAC support came from many circles, including feminists and other pro-choice supporters such as David Norris and Bernadette Devlin McAliskey but also including many who believed that the amendment was unnecessarily politically divisive. An editorial in the *Irish Times* on August 30, 1983, entitled "The Second Partitioning of Ireland," made it clear that the anti-abortion amendment was a symbolic reinforcement of the border between North and South: "The First Partitioning we had to accept under the threat of 'immediate and terrible war.' The second has been made possible by Leinster House politicians, led by Garret FitzGerald and C. J. Haughey. We cannot blame anyone else this time. Not the British, not the Unionists; we cannot blame the Irish either—just the Twenty-Six County lot. . . . What we are working at now is freedom from the Six Counties, freedom from the promises down the generations" (quoted in Hesketh, 334–35). The Irish Protestant response to the amendment suggested that the amendment was unnecessarily divisive and not conducive to protecting the lives of the unborn. The Irish Council of Churches, the Church of Ireland, the Presbyterian Church of Ireland, the Religious Society of Friends, the Methodist Church of Ireland, the Irish District of the Moravian Church, and the Salvation Army all issued statements suggesting that the amendment was unnecessary; and some, not surprisingly, made reference to the issue of the North (Hesketh, 385–90).

As Hesketh points out, doctrinal differences existed, but the churches, Catholic and Protestant, did have a history of working together in the North against abortion. Protestants North and South saw that the amendment defined Ireland as the Republic and as Catholic. Again, what was at stake in the abortion referendum was not so much the medico-legal and religious definitions of fetal "life" but rather political territorial boundaries. The Irish Constitution purports to cover both "Nation" and "State," terms that refer respectively to Ireland and the Republic of Ireland. But Fetal Ireland's autonomy required abandoning that troubling political contingency, the North, instead fixing the nation-state's borders and securing its agency at the cost of the so-called Irish nation—and, of course, at the cost of Irish women's agency.

That fixity of borders was in name only, as Margo Harkin's groundbreaking 1989 film *Hush-A-Bye Baby* suggests.[23] Set in the North in 1984—after the referendum, the death of Ann Lovett, and the Kerry Babies Case—Harkin's film foregrounds the juxtaposition of North and South, political and personal agency, sex and national politics. The film suggests that the border is only one of many ways in which women are contained. More to the point, women's reproductive choices are constrained by religious, economic, and political discourse regardless of whether they live north or south of the border; women's personal agency is anathema in the context of the perpetuation of political systems.

The political situation in the North permeates the everyday lives of the characters in the film. The main female character, Goretti, is one of two girls in a Catholic family with republican sympathies. The main male character, Ciaran, is one of a family of boys, a young one of whom is caught early in the film with a petrol bomb that turns out to be something else entirely: in order to impress his friends with a petrol bomb, he has filled a bottle with urine and stuffed it with his brother's tie as a "wick." Much of the comedy of the film similarly emerges from the connections between the political and the adolescent. For instance, when at a local pub with her girlfriends, Goretti hopes to catch the eye of Ciaran. Unsuccessful, she remarks that "he walks right past me like he was charging through an Army checkpoint." British occupation of the North here becomes a metaphor for teen embarrassment and the distance between the sexes. After Ciaran returns home drunk, his brother teases him with a joke: "What's Castlereagh Interrogation Center and oral sex got in common? Do you give up? . . . One slip of the tongue and you're in the shite." The joke makes a flippant connection between sex and the political future faced by many young republican men — internment at Castlereagh — in an attempt to mitigate the fear of the latter.

Perhaps the most amusing and sustained conjunctions of the personal and the political are in the scene following Ciaran's appearance in Goretti's Irish language class, where his apparent linguistic fluency affords him the opportunity to flirt with and impress Goretti. Ciaran's actual Irish ability is exposed when, in order to impress Goretti, he tries to outwit a soldier by speaking to him with Irish phrases that translate to "Irish Tourist Board, Sinn Fein, Irish Airlines, Irish Peat Board, a Hundred Thousand Welcomes, Our Day Will Come" — only to find the soldier actually speaks better Irish. The latter interchange, like the joking way the Troubles are generally invoked in the early part of the film, suggests the tension between the day-to-day experiences of the characters and the larger political implications of their circumstances. The soldier asks, in Irish, "Well then, tell me the impact the Troubles have had on Irish social, political, and economic life" — one of the subjects, of course, of the film. Ciaran, whose Irish is limited to basic conversational scripts, government names, tourist catch phrases, and Irish republican slogans, cannot understand what he has been asked, both literally and in the larger context of the film: the quotidian nature of the Troubles has made it impossible for him to think about their impact in a more than personal way.[24] Ciaran tries to recuperate his macho flirtation with Goretti by saying that "I could tell he was bluffing a bit. It's all part of the game. . . . One thing you have to learn about the Irish language, Goretti, is that not everything can be translated." The poignancy of his ignorance is struck home, however, as they walk blithely by a republican mural: "Many have eyes but cannot see." The "game" of which they are a part—sexual, religious, and political—has consequences unforeseen to them.

The same can be said of their relationship to the religious discourse in which they are immersed. Sinéad, Goretti's friend, plays at being a nun before her friends come to her house to go to the pub. The girls in school giggle and stare in the direction of the genitalia of their teacher, "Father Divine," as he speaks of the glory of "accepting . . . God's gift to create new life" in marriage. Ciaran teases Goretti flirtatiously with "do you wear scapulars?" before they commence kissing. And their first sexual encounter is interrupted by a priest who has come by to visit with the family, accompanied by the soundtrack's surge of organ music. Religion is an occasion for play, one more authority for the teenagers to resist. The extent to which Goretti and Ciaran are surveyed by the church is not obvious to them: the priest's visit to the family is merely an occasion for comic relief. The extent to which the church shapes and limits their choices becomes clearer as the couple are thrown abruptly into "adult" concerns.

Their relative innocence is destroyed when Ciaran is picked up in a sweep of the Bogside (Catholic) district and Goretti discovers that she is pregnant by Ciaran. In one scene, the newspapers refer to the notorious "supergrass trials" of the late 1980s; Ciaran, presumably, will be "grassed on," or informed against. Though his situation is obviously different than Goretti's, each of their particular narratives is shaped by the politics of "information." "To inform" has political resonance in both situations: the "information" relayed in the supergrass trials could potentially hurt the republican cause. But so, too, could information about abortion; Goretti's child would only help increase the nationalist numbers, as this chapter's epigraph by Bernadette Devlin McAliskey suggests. The personal is thus intimately and inextricably tied with the political in this film. Goretti remains silent about her pregnancy, telling her friend Majella that she wants to go to the Gaeltacht as they stand in front of the well-known Bogside mural, "You Are Now Entering Free Derry."[25] The mural, ironic enough on its own given the political and economic constraints that persist in the Bogside, gains further poignant irony in the face of Goretti's problem: in no way is Derry "free" for Goretti, whose choices are limited by lack of information and by the moral dictates of the Church.

Consulting her pocket Irish dictionary, Goretti attempts to inform Ciaran of her pregnancy by writing a letter to him in jail that reads, "I am carrying the family." Her euphemistic attempt at expressing her condition marks her entrance into the larger politics of reproduction: as an Irish Catholic woman, the burden of "carrying"—maintaining, reproducing—the family is indeed upon her. This responsibility weighs on her even as she crosses the checkpoint into Donegal; crossing that border affords no relief. Her attempt to inform Ciaran by letter is thwarted: written in Irish, her message does not make it through the censors, who fear that personal communication in Irish necessarily has political relevance. The joking ways in which the Irish language is used earlier in the film again turn serious when the couple find themselves consciously aware of the larger political context in which they are involved.

Once Goretti and her friend Deirdre ("Dinky") arrive in the Donegal Gaeltacht, the film evokes a number of images associated with the abortion debates. They see a grotto of the Virgin Mary and discuss whether its eyes will move. The grotto recalls not only the sightings of similar phenomena around the island but also the death of Ann Lovett at the foot of the grotto of the Virgin at Granard. The Virgin signifies in a number of ways throughout the rest of the film: she serves as an object of scrutiny, a symbol of inaction in the face of crisis, and a screen on which to project the judgments of a religious nation. As Cullingford reminds us, the Virgin statues were said by religious commentators to be moving because "Our Lady was disturbed by the terrible events of 1984," though, Cullingford adds, "on what score?" (48). The girls remain fairly certain that her eyes will not move; Goretti remarks that "I don't think any have moved in Donegal or in the North for that matter, so I think we're safe." Her comment suggests that the Virgin's movement would signal disapproval of her. This reading is reinforced by Dinky as they leave town after Goretti has broken the news to her: Dinky yells laughingly at the statue, "Don't you fucking move!" But Goretti's comment also suggests that she expects no help from the Virgin, who may watch her but who is ultimately contained and immobile under glass.

Ann Lovett is again evoked as Goretti turns the kitchen radio from traditional music on Raidió na nGaeltachta to a forum on the aftermath of the abortion referendum. She changes the radio station as the woman of the house returns to the kitchen; she is afraid even to listen to the station for fear of association with the issues being discussed. When the woman leaves, Goretti returns to the station to listen to the two women on the program discuss the "prevailing attitudes" about abortion. The first woman cites the oft-quoted statement by Bishop Cassidy about the danger of women's wombs; the second replies with "sure Ann Lovett had the benefit of that wisdom when she lay dying in the field at Granard, fifteen years of age, and at the grotto of the Virgin Mary as well."

The discussion only increases Goretti's distress and highlights to the viewer the connection between Goretti and Ann Lovett: both pregnant, both looking to the Virgin, and both only fifteen years old. Goretti dreams of the Virgin statue at the crossroads turned into a human pregnant woman pressed against the glass. The Virgin now signifies how clearly she and other women are trapped in the religious construction of the female: the glass of the Virgin grotto prevents movement, as does the unrealistic ideal that requires women paradoxically to be both virgins and mothers. In her waking hours, Goretti sits watching the tide come in on a shoreline where lay blue fertilizer bags, visual reminders of the bag found with the Cahirciveen baby and also, as Harkin has told Cullingford, the Virgin Mary, whose color is blue ("Seamus and Sinéad," 48). That Goretti, while pondering the waves along a shore of egg-like stones, sits visibly below the high-water mark suggests that she sees the ocean as a means to a permanent escape from the containment enforced by her condition.

After leaving the Gaeltacht and returning to Derry, Goretti follows the desperate path of many Irish women before her. After Ciaran's less-than-helpful reception of the news ("Does anybody know?"), Goretti tries, unsuccessfully, to "miscarry" the fetus by drinking liquor and castor oil and sitting in a hot bath. She tells only Dinky, asking, "If I miscarry is that the same as an abortion?" and asserting her wish that she had cancer. She recognizes the dilemma with which she is faced: any action other than passive acceptance of her pregnancy would be construed as sin, but so too would her continued pregnancy. Only a miscarriage or something as serious as cancer would free her from total responsibility—though, of course, induced miscarriage is still considered a sin and, in the Republic, a crime; and cancer, despite the claims of SPUC doctors, would not necessarily free her from her pregnancy, given the case of Sheila Hodgers. Her choices are tightly circumscribed not only by the Church but by the internalization of the sexual double standard: her friends, upon seeing a pregnant young neighbor, refer to the girl as a "slut." Goretti's own desperation is mirrored in the following two

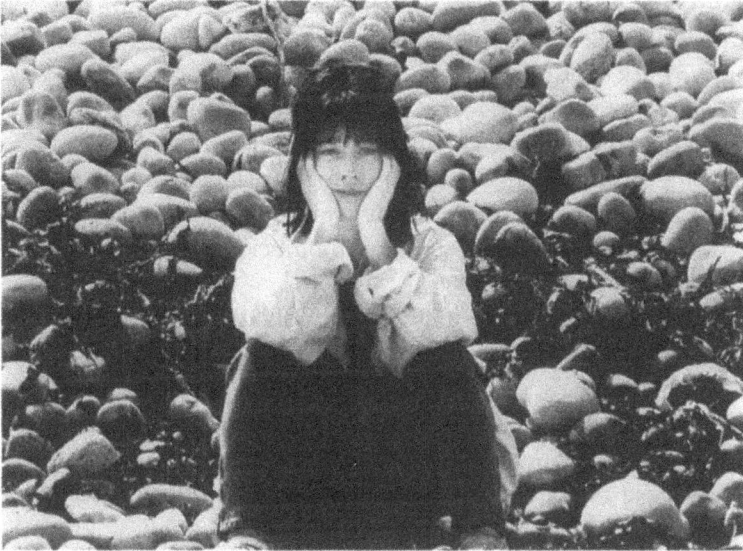

Goretti among the stones (photograph by Willie Doherty for *Hush-A-Bye Baby*, 1990, courtesy of Derry Film & Video Workshop)

scenes. One scene is of a baptism of a baby, a newborn child found alive at the grotto of Long Tower chapel; Goretti suggests that the mother must have been "desperate." This scene, based on a real incident, is quickly followed by a discussion of Seamus Heaney's poem "Limbo," a poem that hearkens back to another earlier case of infanticide by drowning, the Ballyshannon baby.[26] Goretti interprets the poem, too, as being about a "desperate" mother. She turns down Ciaran's written request for her hand in marriage, responding, "I'm only fifteen, y'know." In resisting the heteronormative model insisted upon by the Church, however, she is left few other choices. Her desperation and unsuccessful "miscarriage" lead one to assume that she will pursue one of the other options presented by the previous scenes: abandonment or infanticide.

The latter option is reinforced by the opening scene of the movie, suggesting that the only escape is offered by the death of her fetus/child. The movie opens with an image that, as Cullingford notes, seems to be a fetus in amniotic fluid, then possibly a baby in seaweed or hair, but is soon discovered to be a doll, swirled around in a bath by Goretti's niece (51). Cullingford reads the niece as "drowning" her doll, given Harkin's stated reference to the Ballyshannon baby (51, 53). The repeated images of water — on the shore where lie the fertilizer bags, in Heaney's poem, in the tub in which Goretti tries a home abortion, in the baptismal font—all hearken back to the opening scene and, as Harkin notes, the babies "thrown back to the waters." The relationship of amniotic fluid to water suggested by the opening scene underscores how severely the women alluded to in the movie are alienated from their own bodies. That a fetus can be the same as a child and the womb the same as an ocean suggest that all are seen as external, as the fetal imagery of the anti-abortion groups would have it; abortion and infanticide must thus be morally equivalent.

As the movie draws to a close, Goretti's nightmares of the Virgin statue, now transformed completely to a pregnant woman's body pressed under glass, mix with the visual image of the troubled Goretti as she attempts to sleep. As she wakes with a yell, and her parents come to the door of her room, the last image of the film is a close-up still of Goretti's face. Framed by the television screen, Goretti becomes another "virgin" under glass, without agency and subject to the scrutiny of the faithful. The final image evokes other instances of surveillance throughout the film: Sinéad's examination of herself in the mirror as she plays at being the Virgin, the boys' observation of the girls dancing throughout the film, the police helicopters, the ever-present statues of the Virgin "watching" over the characters, and the surveillance towers of the military. The film suggests throughout that personal agency is profoundly affected by the surveillance to which those in Northern Ireland are subjected on a daily basis—by the state, by the Church, and ultimately by each person who internalizes the gaze of these powerful institutions and begins to regulate herself. This final image, suggesting the conflation of the television screen and the glass surrounding the Virgin at her grottos, implicates the viewer in this surveillance and thus in any judgments of Goretti. It makes clear the extent to which any action Goretti takes, like the movement of the Virgin statues throughout Ireland, is shaped by the expectations of those who watch.

Hush-A-Bye Baby thus shares with Bardwell's "The Dove of Peace" the image of women's problems contained, boxed away, or under glass. Unlike "The Dove of Peace," however, Harkin's film suggests that unwanted pregnancy is always already a public spectacle in Ireland, a screen onto which the anxieties of others are projected. By ending without resolving Goretti's crisis, Harkin forces the viewer to accept that every possible end to the pregnancy narrative, every "choice" she might make, is shaped by political and religious discourse. As Richard Kirkland has put it, "The narrowness of narrative possibility mirrors the nar-

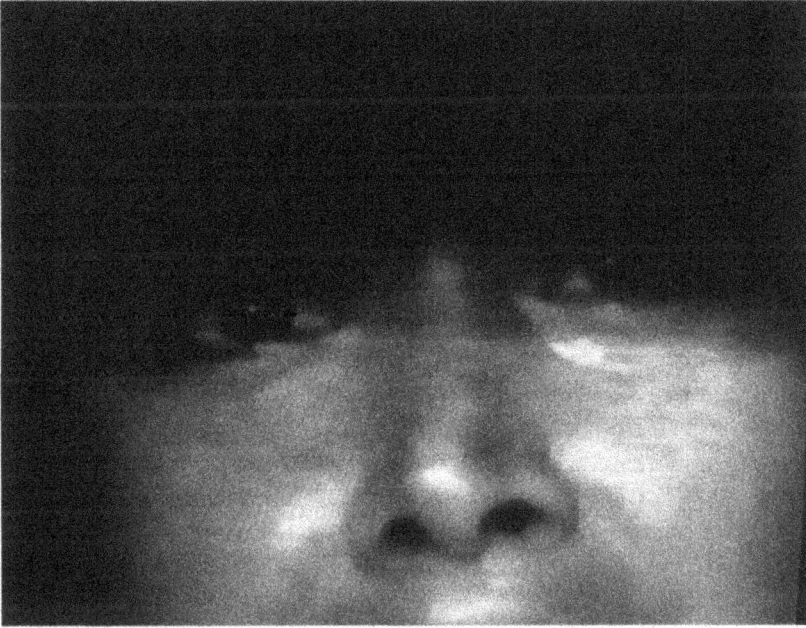

Final screen image of Goretti from *Hush-A-Bye Baby*

rowness of possibility within Goretti's predicament and with this the film's frame of reference inexorably closes in on Goretti and her consciousness."[27] The momentary freezing of that image on the screen further emphasizes the paralyzing nature of Goretti's dilemma. The final scene thus draws us inevitably back to the opening: Goretti has been infantilized, a young woman with as little agency as the fetus/child represented in the opening scene. Not conceding to the heteronormative family narrative and with no other viable options, she is frozen into a static image, forcibly removed from narrative possibility: her face represents the stagnation that results from the mapping of competing religio-political narratives onto women's lives.

Border Crossings: Abortion Information, the X Case, and the Internment of Irish Women

The writers whose works I have examined above make clear, by exploring both real and fictional individual cases, how both the suppression and circulation of information affect individual agency. After the 1983 passage of the anti-abortion amendment, the relevance of "information" became even clearer in light of the continued stream of Irish women traveling to England to avail themselves of legal abortion. The state, while attempting to draw more distinctly the border between itself and the "moral decadence of Europe," only made its vulnerabilities clearer: abortion information could not be so easily controlled.

Maeve Binchy's short stories "Decision in Belfield" and "Shepherd's Bush," published in 1982 and 1983, respectively, speak to the practice that started well before the amendments and continues to this day.[28] In both stories, the main female characters make the trek to London to obtain abortions and face the odd combination of silence and acceptance that surrounds this method of dealing with unwanted pregnancy. "Decision in Belfield" is written from the perspective of a woman, Pat, who faces an unwanted pregnancy and whose sister, Cathy, resides in London. It is not wholly clear whether or not Cathy went to London for an abortion, since she claims that she did not; the characters, like the reader, are left to assume what they wish. By the end, Pat has decided that she, too, will go to London to obtain an abortion on the pretense of working and going to school. The story suggests that London, a site of multiple possibilities and opportunities, provides a convenient cover for family and friends who want to deny the existence of unwanted pregnancy in Ireland. "Shepherd's Bush" is set in London itself: a shy young woman, May, goes to London and faces with surprise the matter-of-fact way in which abortions for Irish women are handled. The story, like many of Binchy's, subtly criticizes the discomfort with discussing sex and contraception that, in turn, can lead to unwanted pregnancy, as well as the sociopolitical forces that ensure such discomfort.

Binchy also raises the specter of the economic side of abortion: "She had once read a cynical article in a magazine which said that girls coming to London for abortion provided a significant part of the city's tourist revenue. . . . When she filled in the card at the airport she had written 'Business' in the section where it said 'Purpose of journey.'"[29] May does not want to be cynical, but the reference to the article makes it clear that not only Ireland benefits from the "don't ask, don't tell" policy about abortion. Ireland exports its problems; England accepts them without a fuss and gains in the exchange. Both of Binchy's stories, written from the perspective of a third-person omniscient narrator, are the narratives of individuals negotiating the silence of a system that attempts to ignore the issues that complicate women's "choices." Both end with the characters still facing the stifling morality at home, a morality that does not acknowledge or address the underlying problems that lead women to seek abortion in the first place: the stigmatization of unwed mothers, the difficulty in obtaining contraception, the silence about sexuality, the sexual double standard, the lack of economic support for working mothers, and so forth. May chooses not to tell her married lover, Andy, about her abortion: "He was very moral in his own way, was Andy" (215). This, the last line of the story, suggests that this story is one of many and is likely to repeat as long as the Andys are allowed to be moral in their "own way."

The silence about the export of abortions was exposed and the boundaries between Fetal Ireland and Europe challenged in an important court case in 1991. A student group made an appeal to the European Court of Justice of a 1986 Supreme Court case, *SPUC v. Grogan*, in which SPUC tried to prevent the group from circulating information about abortion clinics abroad. According to the *Green Paper on Abortion*, the court's ruling established that information about abortion services, when "distributed 'on behalf of an economic operator established in another Member State,' by agencies having a commercial relationship with foreign abortion clinics or by the clinics themselves" could not be prevented by a member state (41). The student group lost the case because they were not commercially related to the abortion clinics, but it became clear that information, when identified as a commercial service, could not be restricted. The disturbing implications of this—that women's right to information was guaranteed only when they were involved with a commercial service—were not of major concern to anti-abortion activists. Rather, the decision made clear that Europe could challenge Irish sovereignty with respect to its decisions about Irish morality, a blow to anti-abortion activists who wanted to ensure that Ireland, like Andy in "Shepherd's Bush," could continue to be moral in its own way. Another blow was dealt to anti-abortion forces in 1992 when Open Door and Dublin Well Women Counselling won an appeal to the European Court of Justice based on the claim that "their freedom to impart and receive information concerning abortion facilities outside the jurisdiction of Ireland breached their right to freedom of expression as guaranteed by Article 10 of the Convention" (*Green Paper*, 36), a decision that was a stronger implicit challenge to Irish "moral" sovereignty.

The silence surrounding the exportation of abortions to England was fully shattered in 1992, however, when a fourteen-year-old young woman from Dublin sought termination of a pregnancy that resulted from her rape by a classmate's father. The X Case brought again to the fore the state's manipulation of "information" for its own purposes. The Irish police were informed of the young woman's intent to abort when the father of the young woman asked whether tests could be performed on the fetal tissue to aid in the prosecution of the rapist. The attorney general was informed, and the police presented the family, in England at the time, with a court order forbidding termination of the pregnancy. The family canceled the procedure and returned to Ireland, where the Irish High Court ruled that the young woman could not leave the country for nine months. The young woman spoke of suicide several times to her parents and to her doctor, but High Court Justice Costello stated that her intent to commit suicide "is of a different order of magnitude than the certainty that the life of the unborn will be terminated if the order [to prevent travel] is not made."[30] The Irish Supreme Court eventually voted that she could travel on the grounds that she was suicidal. Oaks states that the young woman eventually miscarried ("Irishness," 8–9).

The X Case tested the solidity of the borders of Fetal Ireland drawn some ten years earlier. The referendum had ensured a "don't ask, don't tell" policy concerning travel for abortion, again strategically reinforcing the connection between "privacy" and the interests of the state. That connection became even more clear when the X Case exposed the consequences of making the "private" public: the Supreme Court voted 3-2 that a woman seeking to travel for an abortion could be detained under the pro-life amendment. The young woman in the X Case thus had to threaten to end her own life in order to have any control over its direction. The irony seems to have been lost on the judiciary.

Writer Edna O'Brien approached the legal, social, and moral morass emerging from the X Case in her novel *Down by the River*, published in 1996. Echoing the issues raised by such works as "The Dove of Peace," *A Woman to Blame,* and *Hush-A-Bye Baby,* O'Brien's novel, although by no means a factual recounting of the X Case, nonetheless speaks to the impossible position in which many young women like "X" are placed.

The novel's protagonist is Mary, a young woman who is being sexually abused by her father, James, and who becomes pregnant as a result. Immediately and throughout the novel, O'Brien makes clear the problems with the popular and legal construction of the family cell and of "privacy." Respect for the privacy of the family means that those who suspect Mary's condition refuse to speak out; when they do, they assume that the family must be informed, refusing to acknowledge that the family itself might be the source of Mary's problem.

The silence enforced by respect for the sanctity of the family cell is re-inforced by the construction of the narrative itself which, when focused on Mary, mimics her perspective. Although it is clear she is being sexu-ally abused, she does not and perhaps cannot directly acknowledge this; and although her mother and a doctor know she is pregnant, Mary her-self does not recognize or consciously acknowledge her condition for several months. When the narrative takes on the perspective of her mother, Bridget, who herself is abused and quite possibly knows of her daughter's abuse, no direct mention of either is made in the narrative. Bridget dies, metaphorically giving birth to the tumor that represents both the corrosive nature of her own silence and the internalization of the abuse she suffers. Although her disgust about her own condition is evident, she is unaware of the biological source of her illness, since the doctor tells only James, not Bridget herself, of her tumor.

After Bridget's death, Mary is more completely trapped by her situa-tion, but she can never clearly articulate it to anyone outside the family; in fact, she cannot even tell her mother after she is dead, since she is watched by the undertaker. As in both *Hush-A-Bye Baby* and "The Dove of Peace," shame, fear, and confusion, reinforced by the constant re-minders of the importance of respect for one's family, force her into si-lence. She does tell her father, the only person she can tell without risk-ing a violation of the privacy of the family cell; he responds with a violent attempt to abort the fetus with a broomstick. This image of rape is a powerful reminder of the material as well as ideological violence of patriarchal power relations and the kind of privacy they enforce.

The counterpart to this insular and damaging notion of privacy is a similarly damaging notion of "information." Information in this context is rarely shared freely; rather, it is manipulated and exploited to serve the ends of those who want to maintain the purity of the family cell and, ultimately, the national image. Mary's condition is exposed by a nosy neighbor, Noni, who searches the trashcan of the woman who takes Mary to England for an abortion. She finds a flyer advertising the abor-tion clinic and, in a rush to gain fame in her social circle of privileged Catholic women, triumphantly reveals this information to the authori-ties. The authorities are hardly overjoyed when the discovery is made. Because of the abortion amendment, the state has to guarantee the right to life of the fetus, and so Mary is forced to return to Ireland. But the judges and legal authorities in the novel are loathe to deal with the situ-ation, making every effort to be sure "nothing gets out" and cursing the

girl for coming home at all and exposing the nation to its own legal contradictions.[31] O'Brien's judges are a hypocritical lot, indulging in extra-
marital affairs while referring to Mary as a "little slut about to pour piss
on the nation's breast" (190). When they do take on the case, those in
power wield privacy and information strategically, as a tool to maintain
their own political positions. Even one of Mary's sympathetic protec-
tors, Mr. Hennessy, makes it clear that he is "not doing all this just for
you," but rather to engage in a political cause célèbre (225). Mary is described as a "Magdalene versus the nation" (212), but she is only a pawn
in a political battle that she does not understand.

What she does understand, however, is the punishing nature of language itself — the material implications of political rhetoric, personal attacks, and the manipulation of information. She reflects, after being harassed by seemingly well-wishing anti-abortion family members and
"friends," that "words were the things people used to suit their purpose,
to stuff up the holes in themselves, to live lies, and that one day those
words would be sucked out of them and they would have to be their
empty speechless selves at last" (210). Unknowingly echoing the experience of her mother, Mary's words suggest that not only silence but language itself can be a kind of cancerous growth, something foreign and
damaging to the body — not unlike Mary's fetus, created in incest and
without her consent. The text as a whole reinforces this notion, implying
that the rhetorical hypocrisies inherent in the notion of "privacy" mean
that the nation itself is in the process of rotting from the inside out.

Significantly, O'Brien never tells the reader what the judges decide
about her protagonist's case; their rhetorical construction of Mary's condition has already been constructed as hypocritical, artificial, and corrosive. Mary miscarries, never articulating a decision but rather uncon-
sciously and physically rejecting the few choices she has been given. The
end of the story similarly gestures away from language. It depicts Mary
in a gaudy dance club with her friend Mona; she is encouraged to enter
a talent contest and assents to do so, choosing to sing despite her lack of
experience. The final words of the story describe her "song": "Her voice
was low and tremulous at first, then it rose and caught, it soared and
dipped and soared, a great crimson quiver of sound going up, up to the
skies and they were silent then, plunged into a sudden and melting silence because what they were hearing was in answer to their own souls'
innermost cries" (297–98). O'Brien pointedly does not describe words to
the song, and she ends with the meaningful silence of the crowd. By ending the novel this way, O'Brien suggests that the problems in Ireland run

much deeper than one law or another. If there is a solution to those problems, however, it is an impossible one. Although many of the judges in the text, for instance, are represented as nostalgic for a "traditional" Ireland of comely maidens and clear class divisions (e.g., 182, 277), O'Brien's own nostalgia seems to be for a pre-linguistic, pre-Christian past to which one cannot return. As a result, the text ends with a howl of loss, made all the more painful for its permanence. Women in Ireland, O'Brien ultimately suggests, are trapped not only by law, religion, and hypocritical "men of principal" who selectively enforce their dictates (6), but by language itself, a system both corrupted and corrupting.

An examination of the X Case and the dizzying political conflicts that it precipitated reveals at least in part how one could, like O'Brien, lose faith in law and language—and why her text ends with no resolution. The Supreme Court's ruling on the X Case complicated the months leading up to the June 1992 referendum on the Maastricht Treaty, which would decide whether Ireland was to be part of a united Europe. Many in Ireland and Great Britain trumpeted the court's decision to allow the young woman to travel as a first step in bringing down "the Berlin wall of Northern Ireland," in the words of one reporter.[32] But Ireland had not yet decided that the wall should come down. The Maastricht Treaty included a clause, Protocol 17, that protected the Eighth Amendment from European law. Thus, pro-choice activists campaigned against the treaty because it would mean Irish women did not have the same access to reproductive choices as the rest of European women; the anti-abortion activists campaigned against the treaty because it saw the Maastricht Treaty, despite Protocol 17, as evidence of the aforementioned "encroaching moral decadence of Europe," not sufficiently held at bay by the Eighth Amendment, given the outcome of the X Case.

As Oaks notes, "Debates in Ireland over the Maastricht Treaty publicly exposed competing political and social narratives" ("Irishwomen,"16). By "narratives," Oaks means the future of Ireland versus the future reproductive rights of Irish women. She continues: "One [narrative] focused on concerns over Irishwomen's status in a united Europe, and was underwritten by a subtext about women's responsibility to the Irish nation. . . . The Irish government and European unity supporters constantly attempted to disengage the Treaty from the issue of abortion in Ireland, while others focussed specifically on abortion as the most significant component of the Treaty. . . . Echoing the calls of the leaders of the Irish independence movement in the late nineteenth and early twentieth centuries, in 1992 a pro-EC narrative developed in which 'women's issues' were to be subordinated to the interests of the nation" (17). The "interests" now heralded by the government were the economic benefits to Ireland if it were to remain a part of the EEC; Fetal Ireland was thus ready to acknowledge, however provisionally, its contingency with Europe. But that new movement toward linking the fates of Ireland and Europe was threatened by concern over the status of women in that new relationship. The subordination of women's concerns to national concerns is, as Oaks and others note and as I have stressed earlier, a common theme in nationalist movements.[33] As a flyer for the Dublin Abortion Information Campaign pointed out, "If we vote Yes [to the Maastricht Treaty], we are accepting a binding protocol which will copperfasten the Eighth Amendment reducing Irish women to the same legal status as the foetus. . . . Let's not be fooled again. If we vote Yes to Maastricht we are voting for the permanent subordination of women in Irish society, an economic and social situation the Government will be very happy with and extremely reluctant to change." The attempts by the state to deflect attention from the abortion issue during the Maastricht debates emphasizes that women's lives and future reproductive choices—even their status as citizens who might move freely outside of the borders of Ireland—were not of primary interest. Rather, the subject of the debates was indeed Ireland's political agency within that union, not women as autonomous subjects. The former precluded the latter.

Ultimately, the Maastricht Treaty passed. Protocol 17 was designed to protect "Irish morality" from the purview of European law. The result, ironically, meant that for a brief time, pregnant Irish women remained, for the sake of the state, more specifically Irish than anyone else, subject only to Irish law. Protocol 17 ensured, in short, that a particular version of Ireland continued to be reproduced even as it linked itself more fully with Europe. But the "internment," as political cartoonist Martyn Turner deemed it, of pregnant Irishwomen did not go unchallenged. The debate over the status of the amendment led to a reconsideration of the abortion amendment. The government eventually proposed three further amendments. The first, the Twelfth Amendment, was intended to prevent situations like that of X traveling to England: "It shall be unlawful to terminate the life of an unborn unless such termination is necessary to save the life, as distinct from the health, of the mother where there is an illness or disorder of the mother giving rise to a real and substantial risk to her life, not being the risk of self-destruction" (*Green Paper*, 30). This amendment first made clear what

Doctors Against the Amendment had noted in 1982: "Since in the Constitution the 'right to life' is quite separate from that concept of health described as 'bodily integrity,' the risk to the mother would have to be literally one of death rather than standard of life or health."[34] Further, it suggested that women's agency over their bodies was to be further circumscribed; abortions could be allowed in this scenario only if women's bodies were outside their control. During the X Case debates, legal scholar Attracta Ingram argued that the Constitution was incoherent. Accommodation for abortion in Ireland for at least some cases, she argued, "is necessary because a case for some right of abortion flows from every version of the moral and political theory justifying our claim to self-rule (Article 6 of the Constitution); to democratic equality as human persons before the law (Article 40), and the rest of fundamental rights that help assure the 'dignity and freedom of the individual.' This is why opponents of abortion could not trust the Constitution as it stood before the amendment."[35] The government's proposed amendment, then, made clear that women were not to be considered individuals in the logic of the Constitution; put another way, individual sovereignty for women was seen as inconsistent with Irish sovereignty.

The Twelfth Amendment, however, failed by a two-to-one majority (*Green Paper*, 166). The other two recommended amendments were passed. Thirteenth Amendment states, "This subsection shall not limit freedom to travel between the State and another state." The Fourteenth Amendment states, "This subsection shall not limit freedom to obtain or make available, in the State, subject to such conditions as may be laid down by law, information relating to services lawfully available in another state." The Regulation of Information (Services outside the State for Termination of Pregnancies) Act, 1995, clarified the Fourteenth Amendment by stating that doctors and advice agencies could provide abortion information as one available option but could not make referrals (*Green Paper*, 30–31).

The new law was tested in the C Case in November of 1997. In this case, a thirteen-year-old girl was made pregnant as a result of rape and came under the care of the Eastern Health Board, which, following the girl's wishes, made arrangements for an abortion abroad with orders from the District Court. Her parents challenged these orders, and the decision was decided along the lines of Supreme Court's final decision in the X Case. However, Mr. Justice Geoghegan made remarks suggesting that "The amended Constitution does not now confer a right to abortion outside of Ireland. It merely prevents injunctions against travelling

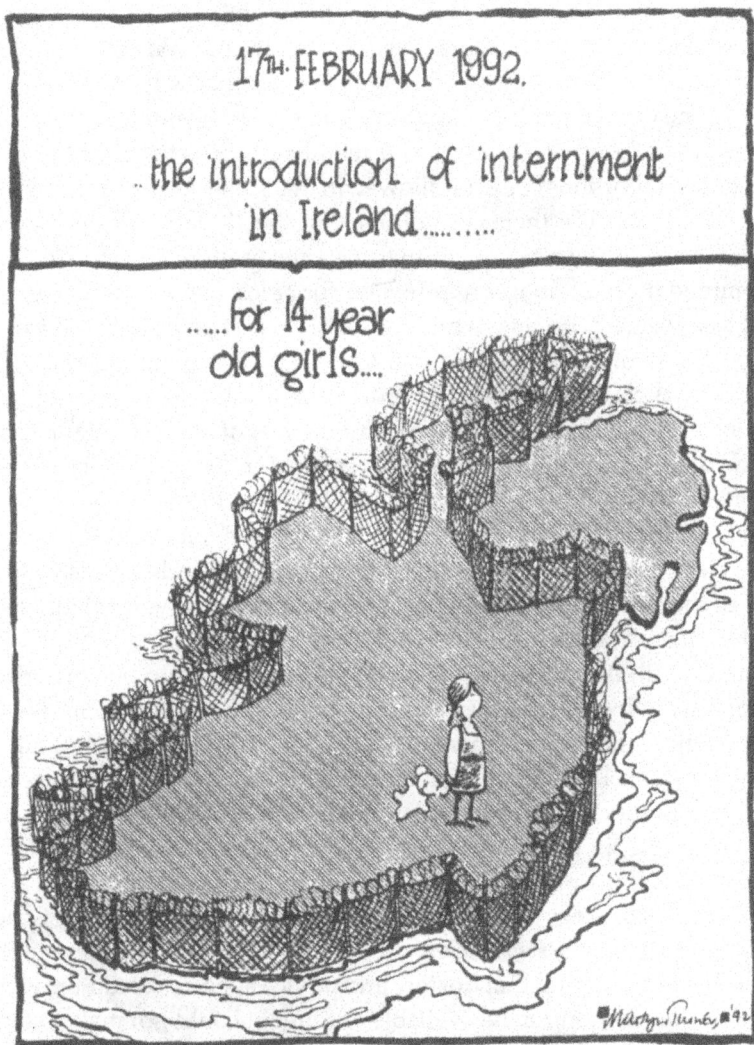

Cartoon, "The reintroduction of internment in Ireland . . . for 14-year-old
girls" (courtesy of Martyn Turner, *Irish Times*, 1992)

for that purpose" (*Green Paper*, 33). As the Green Paper notes, the justice's interpretation suggests that the Court could decide to restrain
travel "by reference to the right to life of the unborn" if, for instance, the
child were a minor—an interpretation presaged in O'Brien's novel. In
short, the new amendments did not clarify the rights of women in rela-

tion to rights of the unborn, nor did it clarify Europe's relationship to the Constitution.

Despite pro-choice activists' failed attempts to bring the full force of European abortion law to Ireland, some decided to try a new strategy: to physically bring European law to Ireland—or at least to within twelve miles of it. Women on Waves Ireland asked Women on Waves, a Dutch-based women's human rights group, to send to Ireland their converted fishing trawler, *The Aurora*, outfitted with a mobile gynecological unit and carrying two Dutch doctors and a Dutch nurse. *The Aurora* was allowed by the Dublin Port Authority to dock and pick up passengers, who would then be taken twelve miles offshore to be administered with RU-486; they were also outfitted to perform surgical abortions but failed to obtain a license from the Dutch government before sailing. Women on Waves also planned to provide women and healthcare professionals with information about abortion and family planning during their three-week stay in Ireland, before sailing on to Brazil. *The Aurora* docked, to both pro-choice fanfare and anti-abortion protest, on June 15, 2001. They changed their plans, however, in part because of their concern about their lack of a license from the Dutch government, but in larger part because they were unprepared for what they found upon arriving: on their first day, the crew reported more than 250 calls from Irish women desperately seeking abortion services. *The Aurora* was simply unequipped to handle such a deluge of requests.

In March 2002, the Human Life in Pregnancy Bill, a constitutional amendment that was the brainchild of the Fianna Fáil government, was put to a national vote. The proposed legislation, which would have been inserted as a subsection to Article 40.3 of the Constitution ("The Family"), would have allowed doctors in Ireland to perform abortions in limited circumstances—that is, if the woman's life was at risk—but excluded the threat of suicide as a risk. Abortion was to be "defined as the intentional destruction by any means of unborn human life after implantation in the womb," although abortions to save the life of the mother "carried out by a medical practitioner at an approved place" would "not be regarded as an abortion."[36] The proposed legislation was an attempt to reconcile the Constitution and its various amendments with the implications of the X Case decision, but in so doing did little to change the status quo. The public debates around the subject echoed those that have taken place in Ireland over the course of the last twenty years. Even were the law to pass, it was clear that Irish women's choices would have continued to be constrained by a confusing, unsatisfactory, and particularly Irish legal edifice. The proposed legislation failed to pass by a very slim margin.

Avoiding the Question: Northern Party Policies on Abortion

The legal situation in the Republic has been highly visible as the abortion debates have received international attention. Despite the initial concern in the North over the Republic's anti-abortion amendment and the applause from some over the limited liberalization of the Republic's abortion laws, however, abortion and reproductive rights have not been a major focus of those parties working on the continuing issues involved in Northern governance. Their silence on the issue of abortion is not an oversight, however, but rather a tacit acceptance of the status quo. Abortion information is legal in the North, but abortion is by no means easily available; the 1967 abortion law that made abortion available in the rest of Great Britain has not been extended to Northern Ireland.[37] And although few politicians will admit it publicly, this state of affairs does help to fulfill an important function: the reproduction of future nationalists and unionists.

Although most parties have avoided direct confrontation of the issue of abortion whenever possible, one of the exceptions to this rule has been Sinn Féin, which, under pressure from their women's committee, established a policy on abortion. The policy has been revised repeatedly, from the 1980 policy, which was "totally opposed to abortion," to several later versions acknowledging women's right to control over their bodies but nonetheless stating qualified opposition to abortion.

In 1986, at the Sinn Féin Ard Fheis, a members' debate was held to revise the Sinn Féin policy on abortion. The previous year, on a very close vote (77-73), a clause had been inserted in the generally anti-abortion policy that asserted women's right to choose. The obvious contradictions in that policy were, as Máirtín O Muilleoir of Belfast noted, a "propaganda present for our political enemies."[38] The debates, however, suggested a wide variety of opinions about abortion among the membership. Many opposed to abortion wished to return to a more restrictive policy of opposition and spoke of the "unborn child" as a life to be defended. One woman from Cork opposed to women's right to choose asked, "When is the taking of life permissible?" and answered "Well, for me, I think in a case of self-defense or in armed struggle";

there was no acknowledgment that abortion might be considered a case of "self-defense." Eamonn O'Duain echoed the rights discourse of the SPUC pamphlets in arguing that "The unborn child is no less deserving of rights because it is unseen, unheard, and undefended"; he continued that "out of sight out of mind is not a moral argument that stands up" and dismissed completely the possibility that there might be a case in which a woman might die without an abortion. The pregnant woman is, ironically, both out of sight and out of mind in his comments.

There are other comments, however, that are even more telling about the relationship between individual rights and nationalist politics. Cuimhin McCaffrey suggested that the move for abortion rights "certainly didn't come from Irish Republicanism," continuing: "I think of the people who are involved in the abortion business in Ireland, and I think of the wealthy doctors in England that come over here, having killed the child in the womb, and that could be an Irish child from an Irish mother, these very wealthy doctors. I think of most of the media that's coming in from abroad, the flashy magazines, and that they are in favor of abortion. They are not Irish republican sources." His comments echo the anti-abortion discourse of earlier debates that suggests Ireland should continue to resist, in Ailbhe Smyth's words, the "global wave of depravity which threatens to engulf it." Irish republicanism is rhetorically posited as the moral protection needed for Ireland to maintain its purity. The difference here is the rhetoric of anti-capitalist and anti-imperialist critique: the "wealthy" doctors and the "flashy" magazines speak to the morally and politically unsound forces of global capitalism, and the English doctors are implied to be deliberately killing off the Irish population, the "Irish child from an Irish mother." As a corrective, he suggests that it would be better to resist the information provided by unreliable global sources and instead to rely primarily on "Irish republican sources." Implicit in his argument are two assumptions: that there are no pro-choice people who are real Irish republicans, despite the very arguments that preceded his own comments; and that information must be controlled by the republican movement.

This expressed desire for political insularity suggests that a segment of the republican movement saw a conflict between individual rights and republicanism. The debate over abortion brought up larger questions about the relationship between the imagined republican state and the individual. One woman suggested that abortion "establishes a purely private form of morality." She argued that the rights of others limit rights over the body: "This particular private morality is based on the premise that an individual has total rights over their own body. But this is not true, for if in asserting my rights over my body I infringe on the rights of others, my rights are automatically limited. That is, my rights are limited by the common good." Another speaker, Dodie McGuinness, challenged this question by asking "Who decides the common good?"—would it be the state, as in China, she continued? For some, the answer was clearly "yes."

And for some, the issue of abortion was quite explicitly tied to the reproduction of the Irish population. Máire Ward spoke to this concern directly: "I think it's absolutely disgraceful that we, as Irish Republicans, are discussing approval for the destruction of the future members of the Irish nation. . . . We are fighting for the lives and the future of the Irish nation and the Irish people." Like McCaffrey, she also uses the rhetoric of anti-capitalist critique, arguing that abortion is "a capitalist means of solving a lot of problems" and an "excuse for the neglect of women and women's needs." Her language reverses the usual construction in which women are blamed for abortion; but by framing abortion this way, she also does not provide any room for women's agency over reproductive choices.

Others, however, supported individual women's agency over the decision to have an abortion. Liam O'Donoghue, a Dublin representative of the James Connolly Cumann, asserted that, "My Cumann supports self-determination for the Irish people. In that support, we are not sexist. We include unequivocal support for self-determination for women also. We believe that women should have the right to decide how their bodies develop during pregnancy and whether they are in favor of that development taking place. You can be morally and personally opposed to abortion and still vote in favor of the right to choose. . . . If people are opposed to abortion, the solution is simple: don't have one. But don't impose your morals on others." This language of self-determination, to which I will return, was echoed by several other speakers and speaks to one way to imagine the relationship between the individual woman and the body politic: each should have agency over its own destiny.

Numerous speakers also expressed the parallels between the current situation for women and the criminalization of political parties and prisoners. Ellie Fitzsimmons of Ballymurphy noted that "from 1976, we campaigned against the criminalization policy of the British government. Today in 1986, ten years later, we are in danger of rubber-stamping the laws that exist in this country to criminalize women who are forced to avail of abortion." She speaks of the British Conservative decision to treat Irish republican prisoners as criminals rather than as political prisoners. She implies by her comments, quite accurately, that the issue of abortion is primarily a political issue. This assertion is reinforced by writers David Sharrock and Mark Davenport, who suggested that, in 1985 and 1986, respectively, "promises [were] made [by the Sinn Féin leadership] to drop the women's right to choose their position on the abortion issue to placate the conservatives."[39]

The decision at which the membership arrived at that Ard Fheis was a compromise. The policy read as follows: "We are opposed to the attitudes and forces in society which compel women to have an abortion. We are opposed to abortion as a means of birth control but we accept the need for abortion where the woman's life is at risk or in grave danger, for example ectopic pregnancy and all forms of cancer" (43). This 1986 policy was revised multiple times. Sinn Féin issued a revised and expanded policy in *Women in Ireland: Sinn Féin Update Policy Document* in 1999. This document treats a number of issues facing women in the North and the Republic, including but not limited to reproductive health, access to contraception and information, and abortion. The section on women and reproduction is quite extensive, citing statistics on abortions performed abroad and polls about liberalization, descriptions of contraceptive techniques and other reproductive technologies, and a long list of Sinn Féin positions. The conservatism of the reproductive policies in both the Republic and the North are blamed here on partition — an interesting assertion, given the conservatism of a considerable segment of the membership of Sinn Féin. Although the document does assert that "lack of control over reproduction means lack of choices in life" (27), it repeats the wording of the 1986 policy almost verbatim (28) and merely states that it "resolves to hold an internal debate on women's reproductive choices" (29); clearly, the issue is far from resolved. As Richard Kirkland has noted, "The issue of abortion . . . indicates precisely where the borders of individual free will are to be found" (62).

Northern politicians' reticence about addressing the issue of women's reproductive agency has by no means been limited to Sinn Féin. At the 1993 Northeast Regional American Conference for Irish Studies meeting in Westfield, Massachusetts, Sean Farron of the Social Democratic Labour Party (SDLP) and unionist politician Ian Paisley Jr. were part of a discussion of the future of Northern Ireland. After their talks, a fellow scholar from the University of Alberta, Heather Zwicker, and I approached each and asked how women figured in their views of the North and its relationship to Ireland. Both of them answered the same way: "We're building a country here; what do women's issues have to do with that?"—although each was also quick to point out that there were women actively involved in their parties. We pressed them further, asking their party's view of the X Case. Farron said that his constituency was pro-life; Paisley answered similarly. When I asked Paisley whether he would press for the full complement of abortion rights, given the unionists' expressed desire to continue to be part of Great Britain, he informed me that that was not a priority. Each of the two men looked to the other for support across the crowded room. Despite their great political differences, this was one issue they could agree that they both wanted to ignore.

In light of the rest of this chapter, their responses are not surprising. Their answers reflect the unchallenged assumption that "women's issues" have nothing to do with the work of building a government and a country. Were abortion as readily available in the North as in England, however, the border between North and South would be continually troubled by women who face unwanted pregnancy and who must currently travel to England. The uproar that has greeted those who have pushed for abortion law reform suggests that Northern politicians are fully aware of the political ramifications of the increased availability of abortion. As feminist writer Susan Strang notes, "The invective delivered by anti-abortion groups against reformists suggests a change in the law would transform the north into the abortion centre for Ireland." Strang notes the irony that, despite their difficulties discussing other issues related to the future of the North, politicians, church leaders, and anti-abortion groups manage to agree on this issue.

Such cross-party alliances are occasionally explicit, as in the recently published SPUC pamphlet *A Way of Life: Affirming a Pro-Life Culture in Northern Ireland,* with a preface cosigned by Nigel Dodds of the DUP and Danny O'Connor of the SDLP. And such alliances are not difficult to explain. Both Farron and Paisley, for instance, could ignore the issue because they rely on the assumption that women will continue to reproduce for the sake of their cause and that abortion is thus unthinkable; this assumption is reflected by Bernadette Devlin McAliskey's acid comment about the "numbers game" of the North, quoted at the beginning of this chapter, a comment that highlights the relationship of "women's issues" to Northern politics and to which I return in the final chapter. In short, women must stay within the borders and breed to ensure that their constituency gains or, in the case of the unionists, maintains a majority. This state of affairs answers Paisley's and Farron's question about what women have to do with building a country: everything.

The debate in the newly formed Northern Ireland Assembly drives this point home. The cross-community Northern Ireland Women's Coalition has not taken a pro-choice stance as a party because the issue is considered divisive of women, although it did propose an amendment to further examine "the subject of women"; that amendment was defeated. As Suzanne Breen of the *Irish Times* noted, "The public gallery was packed for the four-hour debate. However, the Assembly chamber itself was half-empty."[40] Dawn Purvis and David Ervine of the Progressive Unionist Party and Joan Carson of the Ulster Unionist Party were the only people who spoke in favor of allowing women's control over their bodies. The motion not to extend the abortion act, proposed by the Democratic Unionist Party, was passed without a recorded vote.

Ultimately, the abortion debates—or lack thereof—reflect Northern Ireland's desire to remain "fetal"—a political entity unwilling to acknowledge fully its relationship with a changing Great Britain, Ireland, and Europe. Such a desire means that the notion of "self-determination" expressed differently both by nationalists and unionists will remain vexed. In this chapter, I have attempted to outline how women's reproductive agency is at odds with the agency of the political entities known as Ireland and Northern Ireland. Anti-abortion discourse aids the state's efforts to construct itself as an autonomous fetal entity in need of protection from outside forces; it also elides the presence, however, of the pregnant woman in the picture, essential both for the reproduction of citizens and the state. In short, the national self both relies upon and must deny agency to the self that is the pregnant woman: women thus become subject to Ireland rather than subjects in Ireland.

Claire Hackett, in "Self-determination: The Republican Feminist Agenda," speaks to her understanding of the connection between republican and feminist self-determination: "This concept is perhaps better known for its nationalist than its feminist connotations. Yet it must be clear that it has meaning for feminist discourse—self determination as the right and ability to make real choices about our lives: our fertility, our sexuality, childcare, the means to be independent and all the areas in which we are currently denied autonomy and dignity in our various identities as women" (111). Both she and Bernadette Devlin McAliskey recognize the linked history of oppression of Ireland and of women and recognize that both feminist and republican agendas call for increased agency for the subjects they represent; such is the ideal expressed in David Lloyd's essay "Nationalisms against the State," which retains hope in nationalism's "conjunctural relation to other social movements" for its "radical or emancipatory" potential. As I have argued throughout this chapter, however, the discourses that ensure the maintenance of one self often depend on the erasure of another self. In particular, the self of the nation and the nation-state have consistently occluded those of its individual subjects, often merely writing the discourse of the individual woman as a metaphor for the nation — as, for instance, in the oft-cited image of Mother Ireland. Of course, no woman is an island; but until the political groups maneuvering for position in Ireland recognize the contingency of the various subjects that compose it, women in Ireland, North and South, will continue to be merely the landscape of state and nation.

3

Stag/nation
Information, Space, and the Numbers Game of the North

> The concept of human rights is not, at the end of the day, a
> numbers game.
> —David Norris, Irish Senator and gay rights activist

> When the song that is in me is the song I hear from the world
> I'll be home.
> —Paula Meehan, "Home"

In the summer of 1998, the Good Friday Agreement (GFA) was approved by 70 percent of voters, the Northern Ireland Assembly was
elected, and we were given the most hope in thirty years for a peaceful
resolution to the euphemistically named "Troubles" in Northern Ireland. That optimism was palpable until July 5, 1998, when security
forces physically backed the Parades Commission's June 29 announce-
ment that the Portadown Orange Order would not be allowed to march
down the nationalist Garvaghy Road. The whole of Northern Ireland
was rocked by mainly loyalist riots, arson, shootings, and bombings
committed in response to the standoff and to the GFA more generally;
the most notable of the attacks resulted in the death of three young boys
in Ballymoney, County Antrim. Dissident republican forces expressed
their displeasure with the peace process in late August with a car bomb
in Omagh that killed more than twenty-five people and left more than a
hundred injured. Since that fateful year, each transition provided for by
the GFA, from changes in the police force to the closing of the Maze

prison to the decommissioning of arms by the Irish Republican Army (IRA), has been met with resistance and sometimes violence.[1]

As frustrations continue to mount, many are left asking whether peace and resolution are possible in Northern Ireland. But few look for the answers to that question outside the usual sectarian terrain. In this chapter, I turn attention toward the so-called private sphere in order to suggest why the sectarian politics of the North continue to be reproduced. The title of this chapter, "Stag/nation," incorporates part of the answer to this question: informing — represented by the word "stag," a slang term for "informer"—is, I believe, central to the dynamics of Northern politics. As the state and nationalist groups fight over geopolitical and ideological territory in the public sphere, they rely on the literal and ideological reproduction of their constituencies through the family cell in the private sphere. In order to control the latter, agents both of the state and resistant nationalisms have made every effort to control the flow of information between public and private spheres. The result, I suggest, is that women and queers are effectively confined to the private sphere, and the possibilities for nonsectarian approaches to the problems facing the North are stifled — a state of affairs that has led to the stagnation of Northern politics.

Numbers Games: The Reproduction of Sectarianism

Gender and sexuality are not only useful areas to examine closely when trying to understand the dynamics of power in the North: they are essential. As Lorraine Dowler has argued, "In Northern Ireland today the primary role of women remains that of the reproduction of the body politic."[2] Her comment resonates with my own work on women and reproductive debates in the Republic of Ireland; with Lauren Berlant's analysis of gender, sexuality, and politics in the United States; and, more generally, with Nira Yuval-Davis's overview of the relationship between gender and nationalism.[3] The future of Northern Ireland rests firmly in the numbers: though Protestants have a 57 percent majority, this is predicted to change to a Catholic majority by 2050 (Dowler, 78). It is worth repeating Bernadette Devlin McAliskey's comment in the epigraph in the previous chapter: "Unionists must ensure that nationalists don't outnumber them. On the other side what are we confined to — outbreeding them? What are our choices? Either we shoot them or we outbreed them. There's no politics here. It's a numbers game."[4] Women on both sides of the sectarian divide are constructed, through the often masculinist discourse of sectarian groups, as those who must do the work of outbreeding "them."

As McAliskey's comment indicates, that work of "outbreeding" is not considered "politics" in the current political discourse of Northern Ireland. This construction of women's place in the political sphere is more often tacit than explicit, coded in idealized images of passive women articulated through patriarchal church teachings, punishments for women who cross sectarian lines, and taboos about discussing reproductive choices. It might be fair to assert that women have the greatest investment in the peace process — not because, or not only because, it is "their men and children" being killed in the violence, as popular films such as *Some Mother's Son* and *The Boxer* would have it, but because the current entrenched sectarian binary requires women to sacrifice political agency for the so-called greater good of the (unionist/loyalist or nationalist/republican) community. As Rosemary Sales has argued, however, the sectarian nature of the Troubles has often meant that women must put aside questions of "politics"—defined narrowly as sectarian politics — in order to deal with issues common to women, such as childbirth, reproductive freedom, healthcare and child care, and gender discrimination. Ultimately, Sales states, "Social policy in Northern Ireland has both been shaped by gender and sectarian divisions, and has also been important in shaping and sustaining them. Official policy has accommodated to the sectarian divide, even where it has been officially 'religion blind', and many of the policies of the Direct Rule period have served to entrench the separation of the two communities further." She asserts that "politics has remained polarized around community loyalties, placing severe limitations on the development of class-based or gender-based loyalties."[5] This has meant that the politics of reproducing for the community has not been discussed at length, because such a discussion would mean opening the wounds of sectarian division, despite the fact that this state of affairs is true for nationalist and unionist women alike. Politicians, as I have suggested, have consistently avoided addressing this issue — even, as Eamonn McCann has pointed out, when a woman's health and reproductive advice clinic was firebombed on the Lisburn Road in 1999: "No major political party denounced this ominous act of arson in the terms which would have come automatically if it had been a nationalist or unionist or church group which had been burned out."[6] Elsewhere McCann writes that, "In the North, many

Nationalist and Unionist politicians say privately that they are in favour of [abortion law] reform but argue that this is not the time: the peace process must take precedence. That is, we must first sort out the Catholic-Protestant division."[7] The silence of the politicians suggests that reproduction remains the unspoken substructure of sectarian politics.

The issue of reproduction also affects how queers are seen in the political sphere. The causes of homophobia and heterosexism, like misogyny and sexism, can be traced to multiple sources. But both the state and resistant nationalisms, such as unionism and Irish republicanism, remain invested in reproducing their own body politic, and thus they rely on and work to ensure the inviolability of the heterosexual family cell to ensure that reproduction. Even when political parties have held a more tolerant view of homosexuality, politicians have resisted actively pursuing rights for queer people—perhaps out of fear of alienating the more conservative members of their constituencies, but also, and perhaps more importantly, because queers are not seen to reproduce the sectarian cause, literally *or* ideologically.

In the last decade or so, some queer activists have put a degree of faith in the republican movement. But even in the professedly progressive republican movement, queers are asked what they have to offer the nationalist cause. Claire Hackett asks, in "Irish, Queer and Equal," "Where does republican vision find acknowledgement in queer politics? . . . [The question] was explicitly put by Gerry Adams and was also addressed by the speakers [at the West Belfast Feile 2000]."[8] Such a question, like the title of the article in which it appears, writes nationalist and queer politics as equal partners in the political sphere with equal responsibilities to the other; but this assumption masks the hegemony of sectarian (nationalist) politics in the North as a justification for ignoring queer political concerns. At worst, republican politics can share the homophobia of the mainstream. IRA operative Brendan McClenaghan came out in an article in *The Captive Voice/An Glor Gafa* while he was incarcerated in 1992, and in so doing he claimed that Irish national sovereignty was the key to liberation for lesbians and gays.[9] But the response to his coming out indicates that the prison cell extends beyond the Maze. As one unnamed republican source put it, "Republican prisoners down through the years of repression and imprisonment have endured it with a pride untainted by allegations of homosexuality. Now we have this gay rights thing inside the prisons of all places and some people would believe we're a bunch of buggers in here."[10] Clearly, as has been the case

with feminism, queer concerns are all too frequently sent back to the political closet until after the revolution.

The Good Friday Agreement has offered some hope for real change.
But while ensuring "partnership, equality and mutual respect" and "the
right to equal opportunity in all social and economic activity, regardless
of class, creed, disability, gender or ethnicity," the stipulations in the
GFA continue to mean that Northern politics must remain locked in sectarian binary opposition.[11] The stipulation that all designated issues requiring cross-community support in the new assembly be approved by
either "parallel consent, i.e. a majority of those members present and
voting, including a majority of the unionist and nationalist designations
present and voting," or by a "weighted majority (60 percent) of members present and voting, including at least 40 percent of each of the nationalist and unionist designations present and voting," further reinforces the definition of the North as a sectarian community divided in
two (5). The practical result of this stipulation is that cross-community
groups such as the Alliance Party and the Northern Ireland Women's
Coalition must choose sides—nationalist or unionist—for "key decisions requiring cross-community support" (5). The numbers game remains, and the voices that challenge such a construction are inevitably
subsumed into sectarian politics.

The stagnation faced by Northern politics can be changed, I would argue, only by challenging what is meant by "self-determination" in the
North. "Self-determination" has been a part of the language of Northern
accords since well before the GFA—"self" in this instance referring to
the political entity comprised of Northern Ireland and the Republic of
Ireland.[12] "Self-determination" has also been the battle cry of both radical loyalists and republicans, although with different meanings: the
"self" of the former is Ulster, and the "self" of the latter is the whole island of Ireland. These notions of self are clearly in conflict; but I would
suggest that groups *and* individuals currently can have access to a politically recognized self only if they define themselves in sectarian terms.
By resisting such a definition and attempting to participate in political
discourse anyway, women and queers productively trouble that static
view of selfhood. To support this claim, I use real events and imaginative texts to examine the politics of information and the politics of space
in Northern Ireland. The tension between public and private spheres,
manipulated through information and shaped by space, must be examined before we can understand the larger politics of self-determination.

The Politics of Information: The Abuse of the Public/Private Divide

This chapter was originally inspired by an article by Sean Cahill written shortly after the 1994 ceasefire first declared by the IRA and later by loyalist paramilitary groups. In that article, based on his 1994 visit to Northern Ireland, Cahill makes two claims in particular that caught my attention. The first: "Closeted gay men cruising along Derry's Foyle River are picked up by police or soldiers and threatened with outing to their friends and families if they don't become informants." The second: "As part of their sting [on Sinn Féin members in Derry], RUC officers raided the Well Women's Centre . . . , confiscating its records full of confidential information. Since Catholics don't trust the Northern Irish State in general and the RUC in particular, reports of rape, domestic violence, and other crimes are made in confidence to health clinics. Women's activists in Derry were devastated at the potential for blackmail and pain these records could produce in the hands of the RUC hungry for informants."[13]

Dr. Robbie McVeigh's study of harassment in Northern Ireland, published by the Belfast-based Committee for the Administration of Justice, suggests that harassment by security forces (here defined as the RUC and the several forces of the British Army stationed in Northern Ireland), including the types mentioned by Cahill, is a widespread problem. McVeigh distinguishes between sexist and homophobic harassment and political harassment. He argues that "the political harassment of Gay people occurs when they are harassed because of assumed knowledge or contacts and their sexuality is perceived to be a 'vulnerability' which will encourage them to 'co-operate' with the police."[14] That perceived vulnerability can be said to apply also to the women clients of the Derry center — whether Catholic or Protestant.

These claims expose the state's control of the bodies of women who attempt to control their reproductive abilities and, in the situations Cahill recounts, of men who have sex with other men. These incidents of harassment are also instructive examples of the ways that information is used to define the boundaries of the state, sectarian communities, and individual subjects. As I have suggested, for one subject to shape and control another, she or he must control the flow of information about and through that subject. The security of the state depends on the control of both information and informers. The state can use the threat of "information," or exposure of personal details, to secure its own self-interest. In both cases Cahill mentions and in the general critique leveled by McVeigh, the threat of public exposure of private information is used by the state in order to extort more information necessary to maintain the borders of the state. The tension between private and public allows the state to manipulate the flow of information among subjects, who remain understandably invested in preserving the distinction between public and private that ostensibly serves their own (private) interests; those who challenge the public ideal of the family cell often see maintaining privacy even at the cost of freedom of choice as their only means of protection and self-preservation. But the private, in the cases mentioned above, operates like a prison cell — not only insofar as it limits individual agency, but also as it serves as a tool of state discipline.

Further research uncovered differing accounts of the aforementioned "information" that productively inflect my reading of informing. According to the coordinator of the Derry Well Women's Centre, officers of the RUC did raid the center and confiscate private phone records under the provisions of the Northern Ireland (Security Provisions) Act of 1991, legislation building on and consolidating earlier acts intended to allow the British crown forces to quell suspected terrorist activity.[15] The raid provoked a general outcry among the citizens of Derry, particularly from women concerned about the possible use and abuse of private records in the hands of police. Although the center has not been raided since, the event awakened concern about the security of confidential medical and counseling records—even though no patient files were taken in the raid (despite news reports to the contrary). This concern is far from paranoid and is not limited to those seeking the services of this particular clinic. As the incident suggests, the Northern Ireland (Security Provisions) Act allowed the police a great amount of leeway in their decisions about what constitutes a demonstrable link between a client of confidential services and terrorist activity. In this case, the records of calls to the clinic were confiscated because the police claimed that one of the clinic's clients was associated with an elected Sinn Féin city councilwoman — an arguably tenuous link to terrorism at best.

Those at the Well Women's Centre were concerned that any further attention to this event would heighten women's fear of using the center's confidential services. Cahill's report was based on the mistaken belief that confidential patient records were confiscated. The misinformation circulated in the press only served to heighten women's fear about their private lives being used for the so-called public good (as assumed by the Security Act). Many of the women who use the service are in search of pregnancy counseling. Though abortion in certain limited circumstances and abortion information is legal in the North, it is by no means easily available; the 1967 abortion law that made abortion available in the rest of Great Britain has not been extended to Northern Ireland, despite the work of several pro-choice groups over the years.[16] Women who seek abortions still find themselves subject to prejudice and ostracism, and women's centers and their workers often find themselves subject to violence and threats of violence from sectarian groups.

Women's centers are not the only organizations subject to police harassment and concerned about discussing it. My contacts with lesbian and gay organizations in the North have led to conflicting reports about police abuse.[17] One member of an organization stated summarily that such abuse did not occur and suggested that my investigation into such claims could stir up bad feeling; another suggested that active homophobic abuses on the part of the police were rare and were, at any rate, a thing of the past, though I later discovered that queers in the community had often reported such abuse to him. Other individuals, however, pointed me to the McVeigh report and concurred with its findings, noting that the abuse of gay men in particular has been allowed under "public decency" laws: gay men are either accused of sexually propositioning other men in public or of participating in sexual activity in public space. The illegality of these actions creates more vulnerability that can be exploited by the police.

The concerned and sometimes contradictory responses to my inquiry into police abuse suggest tension about the safety of the public sphere for women and queers. Both the Derry Women's Centre and certain members of the queer community were understandably invested in keeping secret the abuse leveled by the state, abuse sanctioned under the Northern Ireland (Security Provisions) Act and ostensibly leveled in the name of the "public good."[18] The state is not the only entity that can abuse the private sphere thus, but it clearly has the edge because it is what Max Weber calls "a human community that (successfully) claims the *monopoly of the legitimate use of physical force* within a given territory" (original emphasis).[19] In practice, then, the good of the state equals the public good. The state can "legitimately" use the threat of violence to achieve its ends, especially given what McVeigh calls the "infrastructure of emergency" (24) and the lack of structures of "liaison and democratic control" (37) with respect to the Royal Irish Regiment (RIR) and the British Army. The state thus is the most effective and officially legitimized controller of information in the North.

One can also say with certainty that the state's control in Northern Ireland has at the very least shaped sectarian battles, if not in fact necessitated them. Such battles have in turn spawned control of information, and the often violent control of informers, within republican and unionist communities. These communities must police themselves, and the family cells that compose them, in order to maintain coherence and control. Informers in this context thus include not only those who relay information about the community to the state or the "other side"; they also include those who expose the instability of the heteronormative and patriarchal family cell — the unfaithful wife of a paramilitary man, for instance, or the gay prisoner. The private sphere, in short, is up for grabs in the public, sectarian battle over who gets to control the state, and women and queers are caught in the middle — shaped, often violently, by competing political forces.

All sides of this sectarian struggle rely on the sanctity of the private sphere to create anxiety about the public regulation of bodies: entering the public sphere means "publicity," or anxiety, shame, and ultimately retreat, for those who do not fit into socially acceptable norms. The public sphere thus remains the province of the state and the nationalist struggles that can personally, professionally, socially, or financially afford public battles within it. Those who cannot afford such battles are, of course, those for whom privacy is the most sacred, since privacy is their only protection from public censure — and, often, violence. Privacy is thus ironically both the only protection for queers and women who do not toe the family line and the way in which they remain oppressed, for they do not have public recourse.

Public protection for such marginalized groups has historically been minimal. During the 1990s peace talks, however, the British government, under pressure from the United States, drafted a document intended to replace the MacBride human rights principles (which were rejected because of the nationalist sympathies of their drafter, Sean MacBride). The resulting guidelines, the Policy Appraisal and Fair Treatment (PAFT) guidelines, came into effect in 1994. The government stated that "the aim of the PAFT initiative is to ensure that issues of equity and equality inform policy making in all spheres and at all levels of Government activity, whether in regulatory and administrative functions or in the delivery of services to the public."[20] The guidelines, a sweeping statement of support for public equality, state that "it shall be unlawful for a public authority to discriminate unfairly, directly or indirectly, against anyone in Northern Ireland on any ground such as race, gender, pregnancy, marital status, political or other opinion, ethnic or social origin, colour, sexual orientation, age, disability, religion, conscience, belief, culture, language, birth, nationality, national origin, or other status" (23). In another case of state control of information, however, those guidelines, produced under pressure from outside, were never circulated to those groups in the North whom they would most benefit. Knowledge of PAFT came slowly to groups in the North, circulated primarily by word of mouth. Were these guidelines to be made legally binding, those groups most affected by police abuse of private information and by discrimination would have an unprecedented amount of protection under the law, and the abuse of private information by public officials could be appealed. Currently, however, the guidelines are guidelines and not law. Making PAFT legally binding would be a first step toward destabilizing the abusive power relations that result from the public/private divide. But as long as public lifeworlds and systems are dominated by those who can abuse private information, whether they be public (government) officials, politicians, paramilitaries, or others, the result will continue to be violence, both emotional and physical, against those who are limited because of their inability to freely access the public sphere.

It is notable than even human rights themselves have become partisan in the North. Christine Bell of the Northern Ireland Human Rights Commission notes a tension between the discourses of human rights and "community relations," the latter generally "government-funded initiatives aimed at bringing Catholics and Protestants together and fostering mutual understanding." As she notes, "Cultural-traditions work involved 'cherishing' traditions to foster respect between communities, even when those traditions themselves instigated division and discrimination against the other community and often also against women." The community relations approach, she argues, maintained the status quo in the North, offering no real alternatives and "[denying] the role of the state in the conflict." In response to Bell, however, Mari Fitzduff, professor of conflict studies and former director of the Community Relations Council, argues that "When human rights organizations focus solely on state abuses, and exclude paramilitary abuses, the human rights agenda appears to be supporting a Nationalist/[Catholic] (as opposed to a Unionist/[Protestant]) agenda," a perception that has resulted in the "ghettoizing [of] human rights." Ultimately, she suggests, human rights are subsumed into sectarian politics, resulting in "two communities, both of which see themselves as victims and who see their rights as having primacy over the other community"[21] Although human rights work and community relations work are by no means mutually exclusive, they too have found themselves absorbed by the hegemony of partisan politics in the North—to the detriment in particular of those groups at most risk of having their human rights violated.

Crying Games: The Failure of the Private Sphere

Given that sexually dissident discourse is effectively contained in the private sphere, interpersonal relationships—those between family members, friends and lovers, even strangers—might still offer the potential for change on the microcosmic level. And artistic creation—writing, visual art, film—offers up particularities that, like the case study, can complicate a vision of politics shaped primarily by abstractions. But, as several artists from both North and South imply, both intimate relationships and artistic creations can be informed by the discourses of state and sectarian nationalisms.

Perhaps the most famous, or infamous, treatment of the relationship between the private sphere of interpersonal and sexual relations and a public sphere of nationalist politics in the North is Neil Jordan's film *The Crying Game*. I want to approach the film via what has been cited as its inspiration, Frank O'Connor's short story "Guests of the Nation," a story set in the North during the Anglo-Irish War. The politics of O'Connor's story are defined by nation, class, and economics; *The Crying Game*'s politics, more clearly and famously, are defined by nation, gender, sexuality, and, to a lesser degree, race and Empire.[22] Despite their different contours, however, the narratives share a focus on the relationship between intimacy and politics. "Guests of the Nation" presents us with one representation of the ways potentially revolutionary affective bonds are ultimately contained by national interests; and the story's continued relevance suggests the extent to which the political dynamics it exposes continue to shape the politics of the North.

In this story, the narrator, an IRA operative guarding two British soldiers, Belcher and Hawkins, is faced with a moral and political choice: whether to carry out the execution of these prisoners whom the community has come to treat as "guests." One of the "guests" is, as he describes himself, a communist or an anarchist, arguing against the capitalist exploitation of workers at home and abroad. He faces off repeatedly against Noble, an IRA man whose brother is a priest, discussing the relationship between nation and religion and the manipulation of the church by capitalists. As they argue, they become "chums"; as they become chums, O'Connor presents the reader with an ideal, perhaps his own ideal, of political exchange: the private exchange of opinion between friends, all of whom feel disenfranchised politically or economically or culturally, an exchange that ideally affects politics on a larger scale. In other words, the affective bond and the "hospitality" of the private sphere create a space for dialogue that can challenge the primarily nationalist definition of the public sphere.

But the narrator and his friend Noble have to kill the soldiers when their commander informs them that the latter are hostages. Suddenly, the equal exchange is revealed as unequal; one party holds the gun, the other only words, an appeal to an affective bond, and a promise to join forces if only they are released. Of course, this cannot happen, and the nation executes its guests. O'Connor seems to present a critique of political systems and affiliations or at least to point out the moral confusion when the public (a site for political engagement and resistance) meets the private (the site of individual engagement and affective bonds). The narrator ends his story feeling "very small and very lost and lonely," and "anything that ever happened to me afterwards, I never felt the same about again."[23] The effect, then, is solely on the affective bonds in the private sphere, and O'Connor pointedly ends with affect rather than transformation: the needs of the nascent nation limit what can effectively happen in the private sphere.

O'Connor's 1931 story provides a starting point for Jordan's 1992 film *The Crying Game*. O'Connor's story is echoed in the beginning of the film, as the soldier Jody is taken captive by IRA operatives, one of whom — the female operative, Jude — seduces him at a carnival. Intimacy develops between Jody and the IRA man, Fergus, and as in O'Connor's story, the intimacy is challenged by a directive to kill the prisoner as a retribution for murders committed by the British. The difference, of course, is that Fergus lets Jody go. Jody dies anyway, however, when he literally runs into the machinery of the state: he is hit by a British tank. One could read Jordan's vision as even more pessimistic than that of O'Connor, since the affective bonds here do prevent murder between friends, only to result in death at the hand of the impersonal forces of the state. But Jody has ensured a kind of continued intimacy with Fergus triangulated through Dil, Jody's transgendered lover, whose welfare Jody has entrusted to Fergus. The film thus holds out the hope that, once outside the confines of the North, the intimate connection will be transformative.

The film begins and ends in the same way: with the juxtaposition of the personal and the political, the private relationship and the public sphere. The public sphere is represented first as carnival, finally as prison; and lest we believe that the carnival is a Bakhtinian site for transgression, any transgressive potential is quickly exposed as illusory. Both sites are, like the Northern Ireland to which the film alludes, subject to literal surveillance, whether it be by revolutionary Irish nationalist paramilitary groups policing the police or by the British state observing its inmates through glass, camera, or window.

The Crying Game's depiction of the embattled public sphere seems chillingly accurate. The film's hopes seem to lie with the private sphere, the sphere of individual human relationships. In this film, the public is where gender and sexual norms and stereotypes are reinforced, even when they are threatening or personally damaging; the private sphere is the only space where alternatives can be explored. The public sphere of politics is full of falsehoods and deceptions and violence. The film reinforces some of the attitudes about the place of gender and sexuality in the public sphere while at the same time pointing at least obliquely to the dangers of this view. That is, while Dil might be safe with her Jody, and Dil might eventually be safe with his Fergus, the private relationship is not so distinct from or safe from the public; the state and those looking to establish a new nation-state intrude at uncontrollable moments. The threat of informing continually troubles any comfort the characters experience: Dil fears that her transgendered status will be exposed to Fergus too early; Fergus fears his relationship with Dil will be exposed to anyone; Jude, aware of the latter relationship, fears that Fergus is unreliable and will inform on her IRA cell. Baroness Gaitskell's comments echo here: nation-states, both established and potential, are shaped by informers. And here the Irish Republican revolutionary cell does as much if not more policing than the British. The queerest characters are, ironically, safest in the literal prison with which the film ends.

The film suggests the extent to which the Northern Irish public sphere is shaped, as it was in O'Connor's time, primarily by a single definition of the public: nationalist politics. This construction of the public is echoed in Northern writer Stephen Birkett's 1999 novel, *Ulster Alien.* The book is described as "a poignant coming-out story set amidst the troubles of Northern Ireland." The back cover, which pitches the book to potential readers, frames the novel as a Bildungsroman: "Meet Matthew Woodhead — a sensitive child with his beloved best friend Danny; an awkward teenager struggling to fit in with the gang; a young gay man on the brink of coming out. But in Northern Ireland everything is more complicated. Matthew's journey to adulthood takes place against a background of civil rights protests, terrorist bombings and the Save Ulster from Sodomy campaign. A world where young lives are destroyed by murder, and young minds by sectarian bigotry. Closely modelled on his own experience, Stephen Birkett portrays a world where the bonds of male friendship are strong, but a gay identity is that much harder to attain." The cover description accurately sets forth the major concerns of the novel: this is a romance as well as a Bildungsroman, and the politics of Northern Ireland are indeed a backdrop; they are not the center of the text. But they also importantly shape the character's sexuality. Matthew is a Protestant and initially and for some time naive in his privilege; he learns about politics through his emotional attachment to Danny, his working-class Catholic friend whose family is caught in the middle of sectarian fighting in Derry. His developing love interest is Alex, a friend who as young man joins the RUC. Matthew resists telling Alex of his emerging sexual identity, however, because he fears police recriminations as much as personal ones, particularly heightened in the late 1970s during the RUC raids on homosexuals. While elements of the text are fictionalized, Birkett uses the real backdrop of events as a guide, including the civil rights battles of the 1960s, Jeff Dudgeon's case in the 1970s — Dudgeon even appears as a character — and Paisley's "Save Ulster from Sodomy" campaign.

As with the other texts examined above, faith here is placed in the private sphere. Matthew's emerging identity is accepted, in varying degrees, by all of his friends and eventually by his family; his identity can coexist alongside the heterosexual family cell. The last scenes, however, in which Alex himself comes to terms with his desire for Matthew, are unusual in form. The narration, in the third person and limited to Matthew throughout, briefly and penultimately switches to Alex as Alex realizes "the beautiful man before him" and recognizes that he "had never felt like this before." This move away from Matthew's perspective is a jarring moment in the text. One might simply dismiss this as bad writing, of course, but I would argue that the implications of the final pages point toward a resolution outside the narrative and outside Matthew. The narrative switches back to Matthew in the final lines: "Game, set, and match, he thought as he sank into Alex's arms."[24]

What is the game here? The game of love, presumably, that crying game to which Jordan alludes in his film's title. This narrative appears to have a happy ending, to be a feel-good romance. The author's need to go into Alex's head before that final "game call," however, suggests strongly that the "game" cannot be won by Matthew; this implies that we as readers need confirmation from this police officer that he shares the affective bond, that he is neither going to turn Matthew out or turn him in, inform on him. We cannot trust Matthew even to see it in his eyes, or feel it in the embrace, as is often the convention in the romance. The choice, in other words, is not with him, as mature and confident as he is by the end of the novel. Whether or not Birkett intends it, the ending troubles the happy resolution of the narrative. The novel reveals that the forces dominating the public sphere limit not only private actions but even extend into imaginative space.

Each of these narratives, then, working in slightly different modes, contexts, and times, first presents the private, affective bond as the only hope for challenging the state of affairs in the public sphere and then effectively undermines that hope. As texts, Jordan's film and Birkett's novel may hold out the hope that their audiences might be moved, and that this affective response in individuals may in turn eventually lead to change—in other words, the texts potentially mediate between the private and public spheres. But there is a certain amount of containment already operating in both cases. Jordan's film has entered the popular imagination, but generally as a gender "whodunit" in which the climax is the revelation of Dil's penis and "real" gender/sexual identity; the conversation has thus tended to focus on the film's negotiation of adopted and "essential" identities rather than in its negotiation of political space and place. Birkett's novel, on the other hand, is framed by the book jacket description and by the fact that it is published by Gay Men's Press. It may well gain an international readership, but the question remains whether it will make an impact outside of an already queer and queer-friendly community.

While artists attempt to articulate the relationship between private intimacies and public politics in imaginative space, those groups who define themselves in terms outside sectarian language have tried to find respite in other spaces in Northern Ireland. Women and queers in particular, groups that potentially threaten the secure reproduction of the sectarian politics of the North, have both tried to articulate theoretical space and secure physical space in which they can be "themselves"— acts that are in themselves politically challenging. The concept of space, like the concept of information, is essential to understanding the politics of selfhood in Northern Ireland. Selves or subjects do not exist only as abstract concepts: they require space. The next section thus engages briefly with "space" and its role in shaping political agency in the North.

The Politics of Space: Locked in the Private Cell

Space is highly politicized in Northern Ireland — a place where sectarian community borders are marked by curbs painted in the flag of the nation to which a given community pledges allegiance or by wall murals that invoke static histories of community triumphs and oppressions; where skirmishes are fought over stretches of road down which one community wishes to march and which another claims as its own; where religious and ethnic differences are still sometimes pseudo-scientifically "measured" by the distance between a person's eyes; and where surveillance cameras and security outposts watch over large segments of the population.[25] Political and (para)military battles are often fought over space, both who occupies it and who controls it. Space can be seen as another manifestation of the numbers game. If you have the numbers, you have the space, and vice versa. In short, space is territory, and territory in Northern Ireland is primarily a geopolitical concept, marked by actual physical boundaries.

These are the spaces that are discussed in Northern Ireland and that dominate media presentations of the province. Other spaces — sometimes quite tangible, sometimes more abstract — are rarely commented upon publicly. The parceling out of territory along sectarian lines has often meant little space for communities or individuals that do not define themselves along those lines. Literal space is defined and constrained by sectarian and state informing, as suggested above; the threat of exposure of private "shame" means that women and queers have been pushed back into the private sphere and private space. But private space is by no means neutral or safe, as those burned out of their homes or driven from their neighborhoods can attest.

Fiona Barr's short story "The Wall Reader" is a powerful evocation of the ways that the public politics of the North invade not only the private sphere and intimate relations but also private space. The protagonist of the story, Mary, is the "wall reader" of the title, an "ordinary" housewife in her own estimation. Despite the routine of her existence in the home, she finds pleasure and release in her daily walk through Catholic West Belfast during which she reads the graffiti and murals inscribed on the walls there. Her attitude toward the material she reads is at first cynical; she imagines "groups of boys huddled around a paint tin daubing the walls with tired political slogans and clichés." But she also recognizes the power of the words, quoted often by journalists; "the brush," she thinks, "is mightier than the bomb."[26] However innocently, she implies an important connection between language and violence. Each has the potential to challenge power, but the "might" of language in this equation is potentially even more destructive than that of military hardware, as she discovers over the course of the story.

Despite her sensitivity to the clichéd nature of the language of the walls, she also believes that "a whole range of human emotions splayed itself with persistent anarchy on the walls." She imagines herself to be breaking taboos imposed on middle-class women: "Respectable housewives don't read walls!" But she also hopes to find her own value represented on the walls, "declaring her existence worthwhile" (47). The walls, in other words, not only shape and reflect partisan discourse; for her, they publish intimacies and personal truths. Juxtaposed with her own routine existence, the walls seem to provide the potential for public recognition for someone confined to the private sphere and, quite often, to private space.

The public sphere in the text is represented primarily in spatial terms: the public accessible to Mary is the discourse that is represented on the walls. Her interactions with others outside her home are defined by barely masked sexual violence that implicitly or explicitly limits her movement: the car jacker who shows "the revolver under his anorak"; the loyalists "jigging and taunting every July, almost sexual in their arrogance and hatred"; and the young soldiers whose rifles "lounged lovingly and relaxed in the arms of their men" (46). Both crime and politics are written as frustrated sexuality projected into the public sphere and public space. Despite her recognition of the potential violence of these encounters, the sexual charge seems to her innocent enough; it merely provides an opportunity for her to transgress the boundaries of respectability internally.

When her transgression becomes audible, however, she finds herself materially threatened. On one of her walks, Mary settles into a park bench and strikes up a conversation with an English soldier, unseen in his gun turret. Their conversation is "innocent" (48), confined initially to descriptions of children and declarations of parental affection. The communication continues over the course of several weeks, each of them disclosing more information, more details about their lives and aspirations. One day, however, Mary's husband comes home and leads her outside. On the wall, in huge accusatory letters, the word "TOUT" has been painted. She has been branded as an informer, a spy, presumably by those who witnessed the communication between her and the English soldier or by those further up in the chain of informing. Her earlier desire to see intimate truths published is destroyed by the sectarian politics that shape such intimacies to their own ends. She and her husband are forced to move in the dead of night. Their house is later occupied by "ordinary people, living a self-contained life, worrying over finance and babies, promotion and gossip." Unlike Mary, however, the woman in this couple contains herself in the family cell. There is no potential for dissidence: she is "not the least inclined to wall-reading" (52).

Barr's story makes the constraints imposed by the dual forces of family and sectarian politics tangible. Her protagonist steps outside the family cell and tentatively connects with someone who does not share her community's political allegiances, but in so doing she finds her community to be a prison cell. The walls are not liberatory; the language on them is even more palpably limiting than the walls on which they are written. And their power comes not only from their relationship to the sectarian politics they voice but also from their anonymity and their power to make the private public. Barr's story mirrors the walls of Northern Ireland: graffiti names, accuses, exposes, empowered by the community's expectations for proper private as well as public behavior. The individual subject must regulate himself or herself, for as the story suggests, he or she is constantly under surveillance. To challenge the reproduction of this state of affairs, particularly alone, is dangerous.

The story reveals the isolation of cells, the "self-contained" units in which the status quo is reproduced. Each family must watch out for its own interests and secure its own safety, however tenuous. Those who step outside those cells are encouraged to step right back in, to return to the seeming safety of anonymity and privacy. But, of course, that safety is an illusion, for privacy is an illusion; privacy is allowed only insofar as it reproduces politics as usual.

Many women and queers in Northern Ireland have recognized that the family cell does not offer even the illusion of safety. But those who have found the strength, through organizing, to enter the public sphere have found literal space severely limited, constrained by the pressures of sectarianism on one side and economics on another. The mapping of the North along the sectarian lines that Barr describes—the communities shaped by history and economics and defined by sectarian loyal-

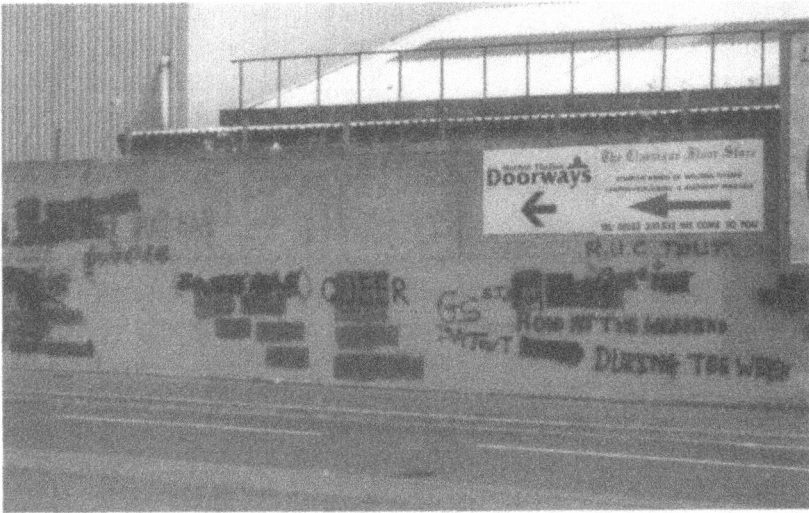

Graffiti, West Belfast, 2000 (photo by author)

ties—has left little "neutral" space for those who do not define themselves in sectarian terms. Capital is concentrated in those neutral spaces,
and they are at a premium for continued economic development and investment: tourism, industry, service, and retail require "peace" for successful transactions; investment does not tolerate violence. Without economic clout, nonsectarian and noncommercial groups must vie for the
remaining affordable "neutral" spaces, even when those spaces are not
ideally located or maintained.

The Downtown Women's Centre in Belfast, for example, is a single
building that houses a number of cross-community women's organizations, including Women Into Politics, an initiative that is attempting to
get more women participating in the public sphere; Women's News, a
cooperative that prints the feminist monthly of the same name; and the
Women's Support Network, which coordinates and serves as a "neutral
space" for various community women's centers around Belfast.[27] All the
projects housed in the Women's Centre work to provide a space for
women to voice their concerns outside the territorialized communities
in which they are often, literally and figuratively, contained. The Downtown Women's Centre is in what is considered to be a geographically
"neutral space"—that is, a space not defined by sectarian loyalties. As a
result, women feel freer to voice their concerns about issues that would
be more contentious in their own community centers, issues such as

abortion, for instance, or cross-community programs. The end of the Women's Centre's lease in 1998, however, led to concern about the continued viability and effectiveness of the groups; the business development of the city meant that new, affordable neutral space might have been difficult to secure. Most inexpensive real estate is located in the more financially depressed sectarian spaces of the city, the very spaces from which women often need respite and in which they often find themselves quite literally under siege. Although the center maintained its lease, its hold over that physical space, a space in which a more theoretical and potentially borderless "feminist space" can flourish, is clearly unstable.

The queer community has also found it difficult to secure physical space, even in the city. As Carola Speth of *Women's News* has put it, Belfast is "a city which doesn't offer much for gay people" in terms of space. This was partially remedied in 1998 by the formation of Queer-Space, a grassroots-funded collective "space maintained by & for the community—OUR COMMUNITY."[28] The community to which this early QueerSpace Mission Statement refers is the lesbian, gay, bisexual, transgender (LGBT) community, but QueerSpace also aimed to "make sure it stays open, accessible, and known both to the LGBT community AND the general/mainstream population," and the QueerSpace Policy document of that period states that "Queer Space rejects discrimination on the basis of: gender, sexual/political identity, class, race/skin color/ethnicity/nationality, religion, age, physical ability, employment status, HIV status, immigration status or other aspects of identity."[29] The formation of this space and the reclamation of the word "community" from its often-invoked sectarian meanings challenged the notion that territories in the North can be defined only in sectarian ways.

Like the Downtown Women's Centre, however, QueerSpace has found it difficult to find physical space in which to locate. Its first location was in the Shaftesbury Square area of the city, close to the relatively "neutral" commercial downtown district and the Queen's University area. When its lease ran out, it faced the problem of finding another adequate safe space troubled neither by sectarianism nor, just as important, by gay bashing, both verbal and physical. It relocated in September 1998 but had to relocate again. It is now housed downtown, in the same building as many of the LGBT-centered services Belfast has to offer, such as the Northern Ireland Gay Rights Association and the Cara-Friend counseling line; it is in the Cathedral Quarter, not far, in fact, from the Downtown Women's Centre. But QueerSpace has become more theoretical than physical. QueerSpace now defines itself as a "volunteer-led organization based on collective planning and action which serves the Lesbian, Gay, Bisexual and Transgendered Community of Belfast and Northern Ireland by raising its visibility, supporting its activities, providing it with resources and facilitating communication while adhering to the principals of community orientation, freedom of identity, ethical funding and accessibility."[30] The services it provides are essential to the LGBT community, including several hours a week devoted to "InSpace," a drop-in community center. But "space," ironically, is no longer a defining characteristic of QueerSpace.

Lorraine Dowler, in the conclusion to "The Mother of All Warriors: Women in West Belfast, Northern Ireland," argues that "true political solidarity does not exist within the borders of Irish Nationalism, rather it exists in the frontiers of Irish feminism. . . . We must perhaps try to escape from a territorialized, hermetically sealed cell-like view of human communities" (88). The politics of selfhood in the North, however, make the realization of such a goal difficult in the current political climate. Subjects need space in which to exist; bodies occupy space. And many such spaces, both private and public, are under siege from forces that threaten the very existence of their bodies. Dowler's statement points to the problem of territorialization in West Belfast in particular. We can extend that argument more generally to the North as a political entity. Where sectarian groups and the state clash over geopolitical territory — that is, the spatial boundaries of Northern Ireland — there is violence. But the violence is not only perpetrated on those who choose to engage with one definition of the national self or another: it is also inflicted on those who have no space in which to express their own notion of political subjectivity and no recognized public voice with which to do so.

Self-Determination, Revisited

As I have argued, the recent breakthroughs in the peace process are far from solving the problems facing Northern Ireland because many in the region do not have free and equal access to the public sphere. Access to the public sphere is shaped by patriarchal and heteronormative assumptions; the individual "self" that engages in the public sphere can do so only if it conforms to those assumptions. The public sphere is also further delimited by sectarian concerns that reinforce patriarchal heteronormativity: women must reproduce for the cause. Allowing people to have agency over their sexuality means destabilizing the security of the literal reproduction of sectarian communities and in so doing providing an opportunity for more people to contribute to a more flexible, less oppressive definition of "self."

Information, as I have argued, shapes literal space. My hope, as I have suggested throughout this book, lies in informing on the informers—not informing as defined by sectarian politics, but informing that breaks the taboos and allows dissident voices to enter and reinvigorate a stagnant public sphere. Whether through pamphlets, literary texts, or protests, this kind of information exposes the ways in which state and sectarian forces have limited both discourse and space, but more important, perhaps, it reveals the mechanisms by which they can do so, the assumptions on which their power is based. The discursive space cleared by this kind of informing may offer a space in which to reimagine and negotiate geopolitical space. But as long as the North remains an unexamined numbers game, as long as politics remains defined by allegiance or challenge to the existing geopolitical boundaries and dissident voices are trapped in the private sphere, peace is merely a temporary quiet; it cannot be a process of resolution.

Notes
Bibliography
Index

Notes

Introduction

1. Throughout this text, I use the term "state" to refer to the "political organization which is the basis of civil government" (OED), "nation-state" to indicate a political entity, as in the Republic of Ireland, and "nation/state" to indicate both nation and nation-state. It is important to note that the nation-state is not necessarily coequal with the nation. The latter construct is, to use Benedict Anderson's oft-cited formulation, an "imagined community." I use the term "nationalism" quite broadly to imply occupation of or aspirations to physical territory and statehood and, following Otto Baeur and Nira Yuval-Davis, an orientation toward the future (Nira Yuval-Davis, *Gender and Nation*, 19). This usage allows me to include, for instance, not only Irish nationalism/republicanism but also Ulster unionism.

2. Michel Foucault, *The History of Sexuality*, vol. 1: *An Introduction*, 108.

3. Margot Backus, *The Gothic Family Romance: Heterosexuality, Child Sacrifice, and the Anglo-Irish Colonial Order*. See especially the introduction and chapter 1, "The Other Half of the Story: English and Irish Social Formations, 1550–1700."

4. Jonathan Goldberg, *Sodometries: Renaissance Texts, Modern Sexualities*, 19.

5. The gendered economy of the linen industry has been well documented; see, for example, Marilyn Cohen, "Toward an Historical Ethnography of the Great Irish Famine"; Cohen, "Toward a Historical Anthropology of Work"; Brenda Collins, "The Loom, the Land, and the Marketplace"; Collins, "Proto-Industrialization and Pre-Famine Emigration," 127–46; William H. Crawford, "Women in the Domestic Linen Industry"; Jane Gray, "Gender and Uneven Working-Class Formation in the Irish Linen Industry."

6. See especially Collins, "Proto-Industrialization," 134–36.

7. Ellen Jordan, *The Woman's Movement and Women's Employment in Nineteenth Century Britain*, 43.

8. Anna Clark, "Manhood, Womanhood, and the Politics of Class in Britain, 1790–1845," 265–66.

9. For examples of this discourse, see L. Perry Curtis, *Apes and Angels: The Irishman in Victorian Caricature*; Liz Curtis, *Nothing But the Same Old Story: The*

Roots of Anti-Irish Racism; Stephen Jay Gould, *The Mismeasure of Man.* See also selections from J. A. Froude, *The English in Ireland in the Eighteenth Century,* 1874/1881; Daniel Mackintosh, "Comparative Anthropology of England and Wales," 1866; Joseph Barnard Davis, *Thesaurus Craniorum: Catalogue of the Skulls of the Various Races of Man,* 1867; and other relevant contemporary descriptions of the Irish/Celtic race available at The Raced Celt Web site, http://www.people.virginia.edu/~dnp5c/Victorian/ (accessed 18 April 2003).

10. In C. L. Innes, *Woman and Nation in Irish Literature and Society, 1880–1935,* 14.

11. Matthew Arnold, *On the Study of Celtic Literature,* 77–78.

12. For sources and a fuller discussion of this phenomenon, see Peter Stallybrass and Ann Rosalind Jones, "Dismantling Irena: The Sexualizing of Ireland in Early Modern England."

13. Nira Yuval-Davis, *Gender and Nation,* 19.

14. Anne McClintock, "Family Feuds: Gender, Nationalism, and the Family," 64.

15. Michel Foucault, *Discipline and Punish: The Birth of the Prison.* See especially part 3, "Discipline."

16. See especially Angela Bourke, *The Burning of Bridget Cleary: A True Story.*

17. Although I agree with Edna Longley's assertion that "unionism since the first Home Rule bill has always been reactive" ("From Cathleen to Anorexia: The Breakdown of Irelands," *The Living Stream: Literature and Revisionism in Ireland,* 174) and that unionism has thus "never developed into a comprehensive symbolic system" parallel to that of Cathleen ni Houlihan in Irish republicanism, it still seems clear, as this book shows, that unionism shares with Irish nationalism the idealization of the family cell—an idealization in place well before the first Home Rule Bill. See also note 1, above.

18. Brian Merriman, *The Midnight Court,* 54–55, ll. 625–28.

19. For further discussion of the implications of the sovereignty myth for Irish nationalist literature, see Joseph Valente, "The Myth of Sovereignty: Gender in the Literature of Irish Nationalism."

20. William Butler Yeats, *Cathleen Ni Houlihan,* in *The Variorum Edition of the Plays of W. B. Yeats,* 222. This implication is consistent with the claim that Ireland was conquered "because of" a woman. In 1152, Diarmuid MacMurrough, king of Leinster, carried off Dervorgilla, the wife of Tighernan O'Rourke, prince of Breffni. A year later O'Rourke, with the help of the *ard-rí* Roderick O'Connor, brought his wife back. Thirteen years later, O'Rourke and other chieftains attacked MacMurrough, overcame him, and banished him. MacMurrough then asked England's Henry II to help him regain his lands. Although the request for aid from Henry seems to have been motivated primarily by the desire to regain lost land, Dervorgilla is often invoked as the "reason"—an interesting conflation of woman and land that parallels the way Cathleen is figured. Historian Seumas MacManus notes: "The tradition is that Dervorgilla invited MacMurrough to carry her off, on occasion when her husband had gone on pilgrimage to St. Patrick's Purgatory . . . and MacMurrough quickly complied" (*The Story of the Irish Race,* 322). He goes on to note that "some however say that MacMurrough forced her off against her will. Anyway, when being carried off she cried out and

screamed, either in seeming or real protest" (322). Despite this rather significant "anyway" and the seeming lack of evidence that MacMurrough's request of Henry had anything to do with Dervorgilla, MacManus says that "on Dervorgilla . . . is placed the indirect . . . odium of bringing in the English" (321).

21. For "unmanageable revolutionaries" see Margaret Ward, *Unmanageable Revolutionaries: Women and Irish Nationalism.*

22. Bruce Robbins, introduction to *The Phantom Public Sphere*, xii, xiii.

23. Catharine MacKinnon, *Toward a Feminist Theory of the State*, 191.

24. Nancy Fraser, *Unruly Practices: Power, Discourse and Gender in Contemporary Social Theory.* See especially chapter 6, "What's Critical about Critical Theory? The Case of Habermas and Gender" (113–43). Fraser focuses her critique on Jurgen Habermas, *The Theory of Communicative Action*, vol. 2, *Lifeworld and System: A Critique of Functionalist Reason.*

25. Judith Butler, *Gender Trouble: Feminism and the Subversion of Identity.*

26. *Bunreacht na hÉireann*, Article 41 (2000).

27. William Butler Yeats, "The Great Day," in *The Variorum Edition of the Poems of W. B. Yeats*, 590.

28. All further definitions are from the *Oxford English Dictionary.*

29. "Informers" in my usage includes spies, those who share information across (generally national) borders but who also may manipulate the boundaries of private and public to their own ends.

30. Ailbhe Smyth, foreword to *Alternative Loves: Irish Gay and Lesbian Stories*, vii.

Chapter 1. Foreign Bodies

1. See, for instance, Jeffrey Weeks, *Coming Out: Homosexual Politics in Britain, from the Nineteenth Century to the Present:* "What is apparent is that, as social roles became more clearly defined, and as sexuality was more closely harnessed ideologically to the reproduction of the population, so the social condemnation of male homosexuality increased" (6). See also Carl Stychin, *A Nation by Rights: National Cultures, Sexual Identity Politics, and the Discourse of Rights:* "Fixed and unchanging sex and gender roles were of prime importance, and anything that could be construed as undermining that fixity was constructed as the nation's other" (9).

2. Although the term "queer" is contested in activist and academic circles both because of its originally pejorative usage and because it does not focus exclusively on gays and lesbians, it conveniently umbrellas a number of communities that fall outside the realm of supposedly normative heterosexuality. By using the term I hope to suggest the largest possible community.

3. Kieran Rose, *Diverse Communities: The Evolution of Lesbian and Gay Politics in Ireland*, 2, 11.

4. Rose, 4. See also Weeks, 18.

5. Ashis Nandy, *The Intimate Enemy: Loss and Recovery of Self under Colonialism.* Nandy's argument finds clear expression in the work of Matthew Arnold as well as in the responses to the British by Irish nationalist writers. Adrian Frazier, "Queering the Irish Renaissance," 10–11.

6. Alan Sinfield, *The Wilde Century: Effeminacy, Oscar Wilde, and the Queer Movement.* See also Vicki Mahaffey, *States of Desire: Wilde, Yeats, Joyce, and the Irish Experiment,* especially chapters 1 and 2, and Bourke, *Burning of Bridget Cleary,* especially chapters 9 and 10, for a further discussion of the importance of the relationship between Irish identity, sexuality, and the Wilde trials.

7. See Rose, 22–25, for a brief discussion of the gay community's response to the AIDS crisis.

8. See Weeks, 23–32, for a discussion of the medical model of homosexuality and the ways in which it drew from the discourse of Christianity.

9. See B. L. Reid, *The Lives of Roger Casement,* especially the appendixes, for a discussion of Sullivan's public statements and, more generally, for a discussion of the authenticity debate.

10. Sullivan reacted to Casement's admissions with anything but acceptance. Perhaps unrelated to these admissions, but worthy of comment: Sullivan actually blacked out and collapsed during the final speech from the defense.

11. A. M. Sullivan, *The Last Serjeant: The Memories of Serjeant A. M. Sullivan, Q. C.* As quoted in Gifford Lewis, *Eva Gore-Booth and Esther Roper: A Biography,* 148.

12. Lucy McDiarmid, "The Posthumous Life of Roger Casement," 128.

13. The "Black Diaries" is the name for the diaries that contain some description of Casement's homosexual activities; the rest of the diaries are commonly referred to as the "White Diaries."

14. The manuscripts of the diaries were made available to researchers in the Public Record Office in August 1959. Most recently, Jeffrey Dudgeon has analyzed the manuscripts, related materials, and context and concluded that the diaries are indeed genuine; see Dudgeon, *Roger Casement: The Black Diaries, with a Study of His Background, Sexuality, and Irish Political Life.* Sharing Dudgeon's view of authenticity is W. J. McCormack, *Roger Casement in Death; or, Haunting the Free State.* Angus Mitchell, editor of *The Amazon Journal of Roger Casement,* holds the opposite view. Earlier books concerned primarily with the authenticity of the diaries include the following: H. O. Mackey, *Roger Casement: The Secret History of the Forged Diaries* and *Roger Casement: The Truth about the Forged Diaries;* William J. Maloney, *The Forged Casement Diaries;* and Alfred Noyes, *The Accusing Ghost; or, Justice for Casement.* This is by no means an exhaustive list; Casement has been an object of fascination for many since 1916.

15. Kieran Kennedy, "Official Secrets, Unauthorized Acts," 27.

16. In his introduction to *Roger Casement's Diaries: 1910: The Black and the White,* Roger Sawyer writes that "the parties involved in the diary controversy at this time [i.e., the late 1920s to early 1930s] were united in one respect only: all found homosexual activity to be at least as damning as an act of high treason. . . . Even after the original MSS had been revealed public reaction, especially in Ireland, was slow to change. This can be illustrated by an exchange between a researcher and an employee of the National Library of Ireland, which took place in 1966. Discovering the nature of the research being undertaken the Irish librarian asked whether or not the researcher thought that the diaries were genuine. The reply was given that the librarian would only be disappointed if a

truthful opinion were to be expressed. Disappointment surfaced immediately: 'Oh, no. They must be forgeries. You can tell by his countenance'" (11).

17. William Butler Yeats, *The Letters of W. B. Yeats*, 867.

18. Yeats, *The Variorum Edition of the Poems of W. B. Yeats*, 581–84.

19. Yeats, *Poems*, 582. The original poem, published in the *Irish Press* on 2 February 1937, specifically accused Sir Alfred Noyes: "Come Alfred Noyes, come all the troop . . ." When Noyes responded to Yeats's accusation, he republished the poem in the paper with "Come Tom and Dick, come all the troop . . ." For a discussion of Yeats's letters on the subject of Casement and his poems, see Michael Steinman, *Yeats's Heroic Figures: Wilde, Parnell, Swift, Casement*, 152–63.

20. Charles Stewart Parnell (1846–1891), Irish MP, known first for his leadership of the Home Rule-oriented parliamentary obstructionists in the 1870s and then for his leadership of the politically powerful Irish Parliamentary Party in the 1880s. The most celebrated trials associated with Parnell concern his alleged complicity with a political murder and his adulterous relationship with Katherine ("Kitty") O'Shea.

On 6 May 1882, the chief secretary to Ireland, Lord Frederick Cavendish, and his undersecretary, T. H. Burke, were murdered in Phoenix Park by the assassination group the Invincibles. Parnell was jailed in 1887 as a result of the "discovery" of letters linking him with the crime. Parnell demanded that a committee of the House of Commons investigate the case; the British government appointed a commission of three judges. In February of 1889, Richard Pigott was exposed as the forger of the letters, and Parnell was released. Within the year, however, Parnell was struck with another blow: he was named as co-respondent in a divorce case brought by Captain W. H. O'Shea, a former member of Parnell's Home Rule party. Parnell's adulterous relationship with Katherine O'Shea led to a split in the party and the fall of Parnell from political power. He died within a year of the divorce proceedings, on 6 October 1891.

21. See especially "Parnell's Funeral" for Yeats's view of the "popular rage, / *Hysterica passio*" that brought about the fall of Parnell (*Poems*, 541–43).

22. See especially Roger Sawyer, *Casement: The Flawed Hero*, and his introduction to his edition of *Roger Casement's Diaries;* and Brian Inglis, *Roger Casement.* Sawyer's "Further Reading" section of *Roger Casement's Diaries* (264–65) is helpful for those seeking other sources about Casement.

23. Reid, 465. The term "inversion" was coined by Havelock Ellis and John Symonds as a description of the "congenital" and "natural" condition of homosexuality, as opposed to "perversion," which was a chosen vice. See Weeks, *Coming Out,* 62. Weeks describes the notion of inversion as "a congenital turning inwards of the sex drive and away from the opposite sex." The concept actually challenged the common notion that homosexuals were effeminate or literally more "female," despite Blackwell's use of the term above.

24. Reid, 454. Compare Roger Sawyer in *Casement: The Flawed Hero:* "The 'disease' [Casement himself uses this term to describe his homosexuality] is more helpful to analysis of the man and his achievements than one might like to admit; it explains a large part of the generally accepted contradictions in his life. He has long been known in terms of these contradictions: the imperial official

who embraced the rebel cause, the Protestant of Catholic persuasion, the Northerner of Southern temperament, and, of course, the prude who practiced perversions—the list can be prolonged indefinitely" (145). Sawyer goes on to analyze in particular the workings of the "frustrated mother-love" that led to Casement's many social, psychological, political, and sexual "contradictions."

25. The practices of sodomy and buggery were subject to penalties under the Offences Against the Person Act of 1861, and the amendment to that act, referred to as the Labouchère amendment, of 1885 criminalized "gross indecency." See Weeks, 11–16, for an explanation of the state of British law prior to decriminalization in 1967. Chris White, *Nineteenth-Century Writings on Homosexuality: A Sourcebook*, contains both the text of the 1828 and 1861 Offenses Against the Person Acts and related contextual documents, including selections from the trial transcripts and evidence produced at the trials of Oscar Wilde.

26. Weeks, 156–58. See especially his chapters "Prelude to Reform" and "Law Reform" for a succinct discussion of the context of the reform of laws criminalizing homosexual acts.

27. Rebecca West, *The New Meaning of Treason*, 214–52.

28. See also Stephen Jeffery-Poulter, *Peers, Queers, and Commons: The Struggle for Gay Law Reform from 1950 to the Present*, and Patrick Higgins, *Heterosexual Dictatorship: Male Homosexuality in Postwar Britain*, for descriptions of the press coverage of several notable trials.

29. See Jeffery-Poulter, *Peers, Queers, and* Commons, 16–27.

30. United Kingdom, Wolfenden Committee, *Report of the Committee on Homosexual Offences and Prostitution*, 115. One of the members of the Wolfenden Committee, James Adair, a Scottish attorney, rejected the committee's recommendations against decriminalization and garnered popular support for his decision. The 1967 act (discussed later in the text) was not extended to Scotland until 1980, only two years before Northern Ireland. Others challenged the recommendations in a more liberal direction, suggesting, for instance, that buggery should not remain criminal and that the age of consent should be lowered to be equal with that of heterosexuals.

31. United Kingdom, *Parliamentary Debates (Hansard), House of Lords Official Report*, vol. 266 (1965), 73. Further quotations from *Hansard* are cited parenthetically as "Lords" or "Commons" along with the date and page number.

32. See United Kingdom, Standing Advisory Commission on Human Rights, *Report on the Law in Northern Ireland Relating to Divorce and Homosexuality*, 11.

33. Richard Hauser, *The Homosexual Society*, 28, as quoted in Higgins, *Heterosexual Dictatorship*, 90.

34. Cindy Patton, "Tremble, Hetero Swine!" 149.

35. Rebecca West, *The Vassall Affair*, 8–13.

36. *NIGRA News* (Belfast), June 1976, 1.

37. Quoted in Mary Holland, "A Gay Time in Belfast."

38. "BOSS Subversion," *NIGRA News* (Belfast), June 1976, 9.

39. Sean Cahill, "Occupied Ireland: Amid Hope of Peace Repression Continues."

40. For a discussion of the Dudgeon case and its implications for gay rights in European law, see Micheal T. McLoughlin, "Crystal or Glass? A Review of *Dudgeon v. United Kingdom* on the Fifteenth Anniversary of the Decision."

41. Jeffrey Dudgeon, "NCCL press statement (Background), European Commission for Human Rights, Application No. 7525/76 lodged by Jeff Dudgeon against the British Government," 2.

42. The Kincora Boys' Home was the site of a scandal in which its charges were used in a prostitution ring led by William McGrath, the house father of Kincora—also the founder of the British Israelite/loyalist paramilitary group Tara as well as a former MI6 recruit. Much research has suggested a wide-scale cover-up of the prostitution ring among British and unionist officials. Paisley's complicity is by no means proven. Different sources, including Paisley himself, vary about how much he knew, but some testimony suggests he did know, as Chris Moore has suggested, and the above-quoted sermon seems to provide circumstantial evidence of it. Sean McGouran, however, makes the important point that many criticized Paisley for not acting when he was told that McGrath was a *homosexual*; such criticism presumes that homosexuality is synonymous with pedophilia. As Margot Backus has pointed out, the subsequent investigation did make this presumption, often using the two terms synonymously. See Sean McGouran, "A Gay View on Kincora," 12; Ed Moloney and Andy Pollak, *Paisley, A Biography*; Ian Paisley, "Miss Valerie Shaw's Big Lie Exploded," 1, 12; Margot Backus, "Constructions of Homosexuality in Representations of the Kincora Boys' Home Scandal"; Chris Moore, *The Kincora Scandal: Political Cover-Up and Intrigue in Northern Ireland*.

43. "Towards Sodom," *Protestant Telegraph* (Belfast), 14 October 1977, 7.

44. "Radio 4—On Paisley," *Protestant Telegraph* (Belfast), 17 December 1977, 6.

45. "It's Sodomy Says Paisley," *Irish Press* (Dublin), 21 July 77.

46. "The Gay Rights Campaign Answered," *Protestant Telegraph* (Belfast), 2 May 1981, 10.

47. "Communism and Homosexuality," *Protestant Telegraph* (Belfast), 17 February 1978, 7.

48. United Kingdom, *Observations of the United Kingdom on the Merits of Application No. 7525/76 Lodged by Jeffrey Dudgeon*.

49. Dudgeon, "NCCL press statement (Background)," 1.

50. See chapter 3 for a full discussion of the implications of the current political binary that defines Northern Irish politics.

51. For further discussion of the implications of *Norris v. Attorney General*, see Leo Flynn, "The Irish Supreme Court and the Constitution of Male Homosexuality."

52. Republic of Ireland, *Bunreacht na hÉireann* (2000).

53. Republic of Ireland, *McGee v. the Attorney General* [1974] I.R. 284, the case that allowed contraceptives to be legalized.

54. Republic of Ireland, *Norris v. the Attorney General*, [1984] I.R. 36. All subsequent citations of justices' comments are from this text.

55. United Kingdom, Wolfenden Committee, *Report*, 22.

56. See Rose, 46–59, for a discussion of the final stages of the reform movement.

57. David Norris, Criminal Law (Sexual Offences) Bill 1993, Second Stage Speech, Tuesday, 29 June 1993, 14.

58. See Weeks, 101, and Laura Doan, *Fashioning Sapphism: The Origins of a Modern English Lesbian Culture.*

59. See Doan, especially the introduction and chapter 1.

60. Doan suggests at least one focus of anxiety in this period: the formation of the Women Police Force, a group that resisted subsumption into the London Metropolitan Police Force. See especially chapter 3.

61. Margaret Ward, *Unmanageable Revolutionaries,* 249.

62. See *Mother Ireland,* Anne Crilly's series of interviews with feminists and nationalists about the tradition of representing Ireland as a woman and its implications both for nationalism and feminism.

63. Anne McClintock, "Family Feuds," 77.

64. Simone de Beauvoir, "From an Interview," 142–43; Monique Wittig, "One Is Not Born a Woman," 107.

65. David Lloyd, "Nationalisms against the State," 182, 191.

66. June Levine, *Sisters: The Personal Story of an Irish Feminist,* 135.

67. Pauline Cummins and Louise Walsh, *Sounding the Depths: A Collaborative Installation,* 6. See also their "An Interview with Pauline Cummins and Louise Walsh," 118.

68. Interestingly, Donoghue cites Lewis's biography as her inspiration for further research—suggesting that Lewis's attempt to contain Gore-Booth's and Roper's sexuality was rather unsuccessful. Donoghue, "'How Could I Fear and Hold Thee by the Hand': The Poetry of Eva Gore-Booth."

69. Sheila Jeffreys, "Does It Matter If They Did It?" 24. For a view of Roper and Gore-Booth in the context of lesbian history, see Emily Hamer, *Britannia's Glory: A History of Twentieth-Century Lesbians.*

70. Edna O'Brien, *The High Road,* 56, 185.

71. June Levine, *A Season of Weddings,* 261.

72. Ailbhe Smyth, foreword to *Alternative Loves,* vii.

73. The controversy in brief: ILGO was founded in April of 1990, marched in the Pride Parade that year, and then applied to march in the St. Patrick's Day Parade in 1991. Ancient Order of Hibernians Division 7 allowed ILGO to march with them after they were denied a permit, which ILGO did. Beer cans were thrown at them, and Division 7 was not allowed to march the following year. In the fall of 1991 the Emerald Society of the New York Police Department unanimously approved a resolution to bar "homosexual and other alternative lifestyle or counterculture groups from marching as units or organizations in the NYC St. Patrick's Day Parade." In 1992 the Human Rights Commission sued on behalf of ILGO for violation of the city charter protecting lesbians and gay men. Judge Rosemarie Maldonado found that the AOH discriminated against ILGO. The "waiting list" to which the AOH appealed, saying that everyone has to wait, was called a "sham" by the judge, but she did acknowledge that, although the parade was a "public accommodation," AOH did have First Amendment rights

to exclude ILGO. ILGO that year held a protest march. An alternative parade in Brooklyn was planned and approved, with ILGO in it. But in 1993 Cardinal O'Connor attacked ILGO and threatened to boycott the parades. The Brooklyn parade gave their permit back to the city as a result of O'Connor's protest. ILGO members were arrested at their protest march—as they were every subsequent year. In 1994 the city gave the AOH a permit for the St. Patrick's Day parade in perpetuity. ILGO members were arrested again, but Judge Robert Sackett dismissed those cases "in the interests of justice." In 1995 ILGO applied again for a permit for a separate protest march before the parade. The city claimed it never received the application, so ILGO was forced to apply again. Their application was denied and appealed, and the appellate court stated that "ILGO has no right to carry its message to the same audience as is present at the sanctioned parade." ILGO applied early for the 1996 parade and had support groups organized for afternoon demonstrations along the parade route. The permit was denied again, very close to the parade date; the appeal was upheld with claims that ILGO's protest march would cause "traffic congestion." The 1996 parade was perhaps the most visible, but each year the city has denied ILGO the permit to march in a separate parade, and the appeals have upheld the AOH march over the protest march. In 2000, the ten-year anniversary, support groups came over from Ireland to join in the parade. Many of those arrested were kept in prison overnight, for the first time in many years. At the same time, a parade in Queens was organized, and Irish queer groups marched, including some from ILGO; but ILGO officially asserted that it does not see the Queens Parade as an alternative to the protest, simply as an example "that celebrating all Irish identities together is long overdue." Sources: ILGO online discussion group; *Irish Lesbian and Gay Organization v. Guiliani, et. al.;* Irish Lesbian and Gay Organization, "ILGO and the St. Patrick's Day Parade."

74. I have chosen to focus on ILGO in particular because it was the first gay and lesbian group to attempt to march in a U.S. St. Patrick's Day parade, and unlike the Boston parade, which was arranged by the allied Veteran's Council, the core of the controversy lies between groups that define themselves as Irish: the AOH and ILGO.

75. For a discussion of homosexuality and American identity in the St. Patrick's Day parade in Boston, see Stychin, "The Nation's Rights and National Rites," *Nation by Rights,* 21–51.

76. Helena Mulkerns, "Gay Pride and Prejudice."

77. Sally Stasso and Anne Stott, *Rock the Sham.*

78. Lauren Berlant, *The Queen of America Goes to Washington City: Essays on Sex and Citizenship.*

79. As discussed by Marie Honan in her presentation, "Traitors and British Spies," at the 1997 annual meeting of the American Conference for Irish Studies.

80. Quoted in Mulkerns, "Gay Pride and Prejudice."

81. Irish Lesbian and Gay Organization, "Let ILGO March!"

82. Diane Cardwell, "The Pipes Call and a New Mayor Answers."

83. Valerie Lehr, *Queer Family Values: Debunking the Myth of the Nuclear Family,* 40.

Chapter 2. Fetal Ireland

1. Laury Oaks, "Irishness, Eurocitizens, and Reproductive Rights," 132. In further references to this essay, it is referred to as "Irishness."

2. I prefer the term "anti-abortion" to "pro-life": as will be clear as this chapter progresses, the "life" that anti-abortion forces are "for" is circumscribed by state interests; and to use the term "pro-life" implies that pro-choice forces are "anti-life," a disingenuous dichotomy at best.

3. Vincent Browne, ed., *Magill Book of Irish Politics* (as quoted in Tom Hesketh, *The Second Partitioning of Ireland? The Abortion Referendum of 1983*, 6). See "An Irish Solution to an Irish Problem" in chapter 1 above, and Kieran Rose, *Diverse Communities: The Evolution of Lesbian and Gay Politics in Ireland*, 47: the pro-decriminalization ruling on the case that Senator David Norris brought to the European Court was seen as "'another example of Europe imposing its ethical values on Ireland.'"

4. Republic of Ireland, *Green Paper on Abortion*, 135. This text is referred to hereafter as *Green Paper*. The punishments are described elsewhere, including in Hesketh, 8–10.

5. Republic of Ireland, *Bunreacht na hÉireann* (1945), 144.

6. Republic of Ireland, *Bunreacht na hÉireann* (1997), 136–38.

7. Ruth Riddick, "The Right to Choose: Questions of Feminist Morality," 148.

8. MacKinnon, *Toward a Feminist Theory*, 193. See especially chapter 10, "Abortion: On Public and Private."

9. Lauren Berlant, "America, 'Fat,' the Fetus," 153. Later included in chapter 3 of *The Queen of America Goes to Washington City: Essays on Sex and Citizenship*.

10. Rosaline Pollack Petchesky, "Fetal Images: The Power of Visual Culture in the Politics of Reproduction," 268–69.

11. Petchesky cites Barbara Katz Rothman's observation that "the fetus in utero has become a metaphor for man in space, floating free, attached only by the umbilical cord to the spaceship. But where is the mother in that metaphor? She has become empty space" (Rothman, *The Tentative Pregnancy: Prenatal Diagnosis and the Future of Motherhood*, 114, as quoted in Petchesky, "Fetal Images," 270). Zoe Sofia notes the connection between *2001* and the "cult of fetal personhood," noting that the Star Child is one enactment of the "perverse myths of fertility in which man replicates himself without the aid of a woman" ("Exterminating Fetuses: Abortion, Disarmament, and the Sexo-Semiotics of Extraterrestrialism," as quoted in Petchesky, "Fetal Images," 270).

12. Society for the Protection of Unborn Children pamphlet, "Threatened by a Human Rights Body/Value Your Voice—Value Your Vote." Image of fetus archived at http://www.spuc.org.uk/images/drop.jpg (accessed 21 April 2003).

13. Riddick, "The Right to Choose: Questions of Feminist Morality," 148. Nell McCafferty and Margo Harkin, among others, also quote this claim ("The most dangerous place to be at the moment is in the mother's womb"), which is attributed to Bishop Joseph Cassidy. See McCafferty, *A Woman to Blame: The Kerry Babies Case*, 10, and Harkin, *Hush-A-Bye Baby*. SPUC's Northern Ireland (Newtownabbey, Co. Antrim) branch also appropriates this quotation for one of

its pamphlets, published after the X Case and the Standing Advisory Committee on Human Rights (SACHR) report on abortion.

14. Quoted in Hesketh, *Second Partitioning of Ireland?* 46.

15. Susan Squier, "Fetal Voices: Speaking for the Margins Within," 18.

16. Barbara Katz Rothman, *Recreating Motherhood: Ideology and Technology in a Patriarchal Society*, 165, as quoted in Squier, "Fetal Voices: Speaking for the Margins Within," 19.

17. This language of potential is reflected in the Catholic Press and Information Services publication "The Catholic Church and Abortion": "The case against abortion is profoundly positive: It is that innocent human life has an intrinsic value. This is so because the unborn child is a member of the human community, thoroughly dependent, to be sure, but with potential for growth and development that is undeniable" (quoted in Hesketh, *Second Partitioning of Ireland?* 49).

18. Ailbhe Smyth, "'And Nobody Was Any the Wiser': Irish Abortion Rights and the European Union," 119.

19. Republic of Ireland, *Bunreacht na hÉireann* (1997).

20. Elizabeth Butler Cullingford, "Seamus and Sinéad: From 'Limbo' to *Saturday Night Live* by Way of *Hush-A-Bye Baby*," 46.

21. Leland Bardwell, "The Dove of Peace," 7. Further references are cited parenthetically. The only date mentioned in the story is the date of the death of the narrator's father: 12 July 1946. The narrator has been in a mental institution for many years and is "old, arthritic," suggesting that the frame narrative is set in the "present day" (late 1980s), while the main events of the story take place more than four years prior to the death of her father (7).

22. See "An Irish Solution to an Irish Problem" in chapter 1 for a discussion of privacy laws in the Republic, particularly as they pertain to homosexuality.

23. Although screened at film festivals, *Hush-A-Bye Baby* was a made-for-television drama, funded by Channel Four T.V., Raidió Teilefís Éireann, and British Screen Finance.

24. "*Tiocfaidh ar lae*" = "Our day will come," a common Northern republican slogan.

25. The mural emerged after a civil rights march in 1969. In what became known as the "Battle of the Bogside," Catholics declared the Bogside a "no-go" area for police after police disrupted the rally.

26. See Cullingford, "Seamus and Sinéad" for a discussion of Heaney's poem in the context of the film.

27. Richard Kirkland, *Identity Parades: Northern Irish Culture and Dissident Subjects*, 63. Kirkland's reading of *Hush-A-Bye Baby*, a revision of a 1999 article, shares with my own the sense that the film shows, in his words, "competing, if ultimately complicit, discourses." His analysis of the film is the most comprehensive I have found since I first published the current analysis in dissertation form in 1996. Kirkland's reading also usefully provides some analysis of audience reception in Derry and places the film in relation to Neil Jordan's *The Crying Game*, which I discuss briefly in chapter 3.

28. As Oaks notes, "An estimated four thousand to seven thousand Irish women travel to England each year to terminate unwanted pregnancies . . . , and this number has been steadily increasing" ("Irishness," 7).

29. Binchy, "Shepherd's Bush," 201. Pagination cited is from the version reprinted in *Territories of the Voice.*

30. Quoted in Glenn Frankel, "Abortion Case Touches Nerves across Irish Society," A4. Also quoted in Oaks, "Irishwomen, Euro-citizens and Redefining Abortion," 18; hereafter, this essay is referred to as "Irishwomen."

31. Edna O'Brien, *Down by the River*, 191.

32. Eoghan Harris, "Facing Down Fudge: Now Ireland Can Look Itself in the Face Again," 4. Quoted in Oaks, "Irishwomen," 14.

33. See especially "Occupied Country" in chapter 1 above and Ward, *Unmanageable Revolutionaries.*

34. Doctors Against the Amendment, "Briefing Document: Some Medical Implications of the Proposed Constitutional Amendment," 5.

35. Attracta Ingram, editorial, *Irish Times* (Dublin), 27.

36. "Chronology of the Abortion Debate in Ireland," *Irish Times* (Dublin).

37. "Abortions may be performed where there is serious risk to the life or health of the woman, where a woman has serious learning difficulties, or when there is an abnormality of the foetus. However if a woman is pregnant as a result of rape or incest, or if her health will be in jeopardy by continuing the pregnancy, an abortion cannot be guaranteed." Susan Strang, "Abortion: Whose Body Is It Anyway?" 7.

38. Sinn Féin, *The Politics of Revolution (main speeches and debates 1986 Sinn Féin Ard-Fheis)*, 42. Unpaginated references to the debates from this Ard-Fheis taken from videotape (Northern Ireland Political Collection, Linen Hall Library, Belfast, 1986 PV 333).

39. David Sharrock and Mark Devenport, *Man of Peace, Man of War: The Unauthorized Biography of Gerry Adams*, 244.

40. Suzanne Breen, "Assembly Rejects Abortion Changes."

Chapter 3. Stag/nation

1. The Maze prison, also known as the H-Blocks, held political prisoners; it was closed, and prisoners were released, in the summer of 2000. The closing was almost immediately followed by loyalist infighting and reprisals within the loyalist paramilitary groups.

2. Lorraine Dowler, "The Mother of All Warriors: Women in West Belfast, Northern Ireland," 78.

3. See the previous chapter and Conrad, "Fetal Ireland: National Bodies and Political Agency." See also Lauren Berlant, *The Queen of America Goes to Washington City*, especially chapter 3, "America, Fat, the Fetus"; and Nira Yuval-Davis, *Gender and Nation.*

4. Bernadette Devlin MacAliskey, quoted in Cahill, "Occupied Ireland, 57.

5. Rosemary Sales, *Women Divided: Gender, Religion, and Politics in Northern Ireland*, 135, 202. Begoña Arextaga has also explored the relationship between gender and political activism, primarily in Catholic West Belfast, in *Shattering Silence: Women, Nationalism, and Political Subjectivity in Northern Ireland.*

6. Eamonn McCann, "Abortion and the Reality of Life in Modern Ireland."

7. Eamonn McCann, "London Calling," *Dear God: The Price of Religion in Ireland*, 122.

8. Claire Hackett, "Irish, Queer and Equal," 22.

9. Brendan McClenaghan, "Invisible Comrades: Gays and Lesbians in the Struggle," 21.

10. Martin O'Hagan, "Row as Gay Provo Killer Comes Out of Closet."

11. United Kingdom, *The Belfast Agreement: An Agreement Reached at the Multi-Party Talks on Northern Ireland*, 1, 16.

12. See ibid., 2: "The participants endorse the commitment made by the British and Irish Governments that in a new British-Irish Agreement replacing the Anglo-Irish Agreement, they will . . . recognise that is it for the people of the island of Ireland alone, by agreement between the two parts respectively and without external impediment, to exercise their right of self-determination on the basis of consent, freely and concurrently given, North and South, to bring about a united Ireland, if that is their wish, accepting that this right must be achieved and exercised with and subject to the agreement and consent of a majority of people of Northern Ireland." Compare Republic of Ireland, *A New Framework for Agreement*: "[Both Governments] will apply the principle of self-determination by the people of Ireland on the basis set out in the Joint Declaration: the British Government recognise that is it for the people of Ireland alone, by agreement between the two parts respectively and without external impediment, to exercise their right of self-determination on the basis of consent, freely and concurrently given, North and South, to bring about a united Ireland, if that is their wish; the Irish Government accept that the democratic right of self-determination by the people of Ireland as a whole must be achieved and exercised with and subject to the agreement and consent of a majority of people of Northern Ireland" (9).

13. Cahill, "Occupied Ireland," 53, 54.

14. Robbie McVeigh, *"It's Part of Life Here . . .": The Security Forces and Harassment in Northern Ireland*, 136.

15. Based on a telephone conversation between the author and the coordinator of the Derry Well Women's Centre, December 1997.

16. For example, Alliance for Choice and the Irish Abortion Solidarity Campaign.

17. I have not received permission to quote from these individuals, so I have chosen not to identify them or the groups to which they belong.

18. Compare the evocation of the "public good" during *Norris v. the Attorney General* in the Republic of Ireland (see "An Irish Solution to an Irish Problem" in chapter 1 above).

19. Max Weber, "Politics as a Vocation," 77, as quoted in McVeigh, 53.

20. Quoted in Christopher McCrudden, *Benchmarks for Change: Mainstreaming Fairness in the Governance of Northern Ireland — A Proposal*, 3.

21. Christine Bell, "Principle versus Pragmatism," 7; article includes response from Mari Fitzduff, 8.

22. For analyses of the film along these critical lines, see especially Lance Pettitt, "Pigs and Provos, Prostitutes and Prejudice: Gay Representation in Irish

Film, 1984–1995"; Richard Kirkland, *Identity Parades;* Heather Zwicker, "Gendered Troubles: Refiguring 'Woman' in Northern Ireland"; and Elizabeth Butler Cullingford, "Gender, Sexuality, and Englishness in Modern Irish Drama and Film."

23. Frank O'Connor, "Guests of the Nation," 418.

24. Stephen Birkett, *Ulster Alien,* 239, 240.

25. See Allen Feldman, *Formations of Violence: The Narrative of the Body and Political Terror in Northern Ireland,* especially chapter 2, for an excellent analysis of the spatialization of historical narrative after 1969.

26. Fiona Barr, "The Wall-Reader," 46.

27. Based on a conversation between the author and Marie Mulholland of the Downtown Women's Centre, Belfast, July 1998.

28. Carola Speth, "QueerSpace," 13.

29. "QueerSpace Mission Statement" and "QueerSpace Policy." The more recent formulation of their nondiscrimination policy can be found at http://queerspace.org.uk; select "About QueerSpace" and then "Promoting Equality" (accessed 28 April 2003): "QueerSpace does not discriminate on the basis of sexual orientation, gender, marital status, HIV status, race, ethnicity, nationality, religious belief, political opinion, disability, employment status, economic status or status as a carer."

30. QueerSpace, "Welcome to QueerSpace, Belfast."

Bibliography

Archives

Dudgeon, Jeffrey. Archive (closed access), Linen Hall Library, Northern Ireland Political Collection, Belfast.
Northern Ireland Gay Rights Association (NIGRA). Archive (closed access), Linen Hall Library, Northern Ireland Political Collection, Belfast.
Northern Ireland Women's Rights Movement (NIWRM). Archive (closed access), Linen Hall Library, Northern Ireland Political Collection, Belfast.

Other Sources

Anderson, Benedict. *Imagined Communities: Reflections on the Origin and Spread of Nationalism*. London: Verso, 1986.
Arextaga, Begoña. *Shattering Silence: Women, Nationalism, and Political Subjectivity in Northern Ireland*. Princeton: Princeton University Press, 1997.
Arnold, Matthew. *On the Study of Celtic Literature*. 1867. Reprinted in *On the Study of Celtic Literature; and, On Translating Homer*. New York: Macmillan, 1883.
Backus, Margot. "Constructions of Homosexuality in Representations of the Kincora Boys' Home Scandal." Paper presented at the annual meeting of the American Conference for Irish Studies, New York, June 2001.
———. *The Gothic Family Romance: Heterosexuality, Child Sacrifice, and the Anglo-Irish Colonial Order*. Durham and London: Duke University Press, 1999.
Bailey, Derrick Sherwin. *Sexual Offenders and Social Punishment: Being the Evidence Submitted on Behalf of the Church of England Moral Welfare Council to the Departmental Committee on Homosexual Offences and Prostitution, with Other Material Relating Thereto*. Published for the Church of England Moral Welfare Council. London: Church Information Board, 1956.
Bardwell, Leland. "The Dove of Peace." *A Different Kind of Love*. Dublin: Attic Press, 1987.
Barr, Fiona. "The Wall-Reader." In *Territories of the Voice: Contemporary Stories by*

Irish Women Writers. Edited by Louise DeSalvo, Kathleen Walsh D'Arcy, and Katherine Hogan. London: Virago Press, 1987.

Beauvoir, Simone de. "From an Interview," with Alice Showalter. First printed in *Ms. Magazine*, 1972. Reprinted in *New French Feminisms*. Edited by Elaine Marks and Isabelle de Courtivron. New York: Schocken Books, 1980.

Bell, Christine. "Principle versus Pragmatism." Response by Mari Fitzduff. *Human Rights Dialogue* 2.7 (Winter 2002): 6–8.

Berg, Charles, and Clifford Allen. *The Problem of Homosexuality.* New York: Citadel Press, 1958.

Berlant, Lauren. "America, 'Fat,' the Fetus." *Boundary 2* 21.3 (Fall 1994): 145–95.

———. *The Queen of America Goes to Washington City: Essays on Sex and Citizenship.* Durham and London: Duke University Press, 1997.

Binchy, Maeve. "Decision in Belfield." *Dublin 4.* London: Arrow Books, 1982.

———. "Shepherd's Bush." *London Transports.* London: Century Hutchinson, 1983. Reprinted in *Territories of the Voice: Contemporary Stories by Irish Women Writers.* Edited by Louise DeSalvo, Kathleen Walsh D'Arcy, and Katherine Hogan. London: Virago Press, 1987.

Birkett, Stephen. *Ulster Alien.* London: Gay Men's Press, 1999.

Bourke, Angela. *The Burning of Bridget Cleary: A True Story.* London: Pimlico, 1999.

Bradley, Anthony, and Maryann Gialanella Valiulis, eds. *Gender and Sexuality in Modern Ireland.* Amherst: University of Massachusetts Press, 1997.

Breen, Richard, Damian F. Hannan, David B. Rottman, and Christopher Whelan. *Understanding Contemporary Ireland: State, Class, and Development in the Republic of Ireland.* New York: St. Martin's Press, 1990.

Breen, Suzanne. "Assembly Rejects Abortion Changes." *Irish Times* (Dublin), 21 June 2000.

Browne, Vincent, ed. *Magill Book of Irish Politics.* Dublin: Magill Publications, 1983.

Butler, Judith. *Gender Trouble: Feminism and the Subversion of Identity.* New York: Routledge, 1990.

Cahill, Sean. "Occupied Ireland: Amid Hope of Peace Repression Continues." *Radical America* 25 (1995): 51–61.

Cardwell, Diane. "The Pipes Call and a New Mayor Answers." *New York Times*, 17 March 2002. Archived at http://www.nytimes.com/2002/03/17/nyregion/17BLOO.html (accessed 18 April 2003).

Catholic Press and Information Services. "The Catholic Church and Abortion." Dublin: Catholic Press and Information Services, 1983. Quoted in Hesketh, *Second Partitioning of Ireland.*

"Chronology of the Abortion Debate in Ireland," *Irish Times* (Dublin). Cited from http://www.ireland.com/focus/abortion/issues/chronology.html (accessed 8 March 2002).

Clark, Anna. "Manhood, Womanhood, and the Politics of Class in Britain, 1790–1845." In *Gender and Class in Modern Europe.* Edited by Frader and Rose.

Clarke, Cheryl. "Lesbianism: An Act of Resistance." In *This Bridge Called My Back: Writings by Radical Women of Color.* Edited by Cherríe Moraga and Gloria Anzaldúa. Watertown, Mass.: Persephone Press, 1981; New York: Kitchen Table, Women of Color Press, 1983.

Cohen, Marilyn. "Toward a Historical Anthropology of Work: Structure and Subjectivity among Linen Workers in Tullylish, County Down, 1900–1920." In *Warp of Ulster's Past*. Edited by Cohen.

———. "Toward an Historical Ethnography of the Great Irish Famine." In *Locating Capital in Time and Space: Global Restructurings, Politics, and Identity*. Edited by David Nugent. Stanford: Stanford University Press, 2002.

———, ed. *The Warp of Ulster's Past: Interdisciplinary Perspectives on the Irish Linen Industry*. New York: St. Martin's Press, 1997.

Collins, Brenda. "The Loom, the Land, and the Marketplace: Women Weavers and the Family Economy in Late Nineteenth- and Early Twentieth-Century Ireland." In *The Warp of Ulster's Past*. Edited by Cohen.

———. "Proto-Industrialization and Pre-Famine Emigration." *Social History* 7.2 (May 1982): 127–46.

"Communism and Homosexuality." *Protestant Telegraph* (Belfast), 17 February 1978, 7.

Condron, Mary. *The Serpent and the Goddess: Women, Religion, and Power in Celtic Ireland*. San Francisco: Harper and Row, 1989.

Connolly, Clara. "Ourselves Alone? Clár na mBan Conference Report." *Feminist Review* 50 (Summer 1995): 118–26.

Conrad, Kathryn. "Fetal Ireland: National Bodies and Political Agency." *Éire-Ireland: An Interdisciplinary Journal of Irish Studies* 36.3–4 (Fall/Winter 2001): 153–73.

Conrad, Kathryn, and Darryl Wadsworth. "Joyce and the Irish Body Politic: Sexuality and Colonization in *Finnegans Wake*." *James Joyce Quarterly* 31.3 (Spring 1994): 301–13.

Crawford, William H. "Women in the Domestic Linen Industry." In *Women in Early Modern Ireland*. Edited by Margaret MacCurtain and Mary O'Dowd. Edinburgh: Edinburgh University Press, 1991.

Crilly, Anne. *Mother Ireland*. Derry: Derry Film and Video Workshop, 1988.

Cullingford, Elizabeth Butler. "Gender, Sexuality, and Englishness in Modern Irish Drama and Film." In *Gender and Sexuality in Modern Ireland*. Edited by Bradley and Valiulis

———. *Ireland's Others: Gender and Ethnicity in Irish Literature and Popular Culture*. Field Day Monographs. Notre Dame, Ind.: University of Notre Dame Press, 2001.

———. "Seamus and Sinéad: From 'Limbo' to Saturday Night Live by Way of *Hush-a-Bye Baby*." *Colby Quarterly* 30.1 (March 1994): 43–62. Revised and reprinted in Cullingford, *Ireland's Others*.

Cummins, Pauline, and Louise Walsh. "An Interview with Pauline Cummins and Louise Walsh." Alston Conley and Mary Armstrong, interviewers. In *Re/Dressing Cathleen: Contemporary Works from Irish Women Artists*. Edited by Jennifer Grinnell and Alson Conley. Boston: McMullen Museum of Art, Boston College, 1997.

———. *Sounding the Depths: A Collaborative Installation*. Dublin: Irish Museum of Modern Art, 1992.

Curtis, L. Perry, Jr. *Apes and Angels: The Irishman in Victorian Caricature*. Rev. ed. Washington, D.C.: Smithsonian Institution Press, 1997.

Curtis, Liz. *Nothing But the Same Old Story: The Roots of Anti-Irish Racism*. London: Information on Ireland, 1984.

De Lauretis, Teresa. *Technologies of Gender: Essays on Theory, Film, and Fiction*. Bloomington and Indianapolis: Indiana University Press, 1987.

Doan, Laura. *Fashioning Sapphism: The Origins of a Modern English Lesbian Culture*. New York: Columbia University Press, 2001.

Doctors against the Amendment. "Briefing Document: Some Medical Implications of the Proposed Constitutional Amendment." Dublin: Anti-Amendment Campaign, 9 December 1982.

Donoghue, Emma. "'How Could I Fear and Hold Thee by the Hand': The Poetry of Eva Gore-Booth." In *Sex, Nation and Dissent in Irish Writing*. Edited by Éibhear Walshe. Cork: Cork University Press, 1997.

Doughtery, Cecilia. *Forever Fierce and Outta Control*. New York, 1998. Video documentary.

Dowler, Lorraine. "The Mother of All Warriors: Women in West Belfast, Northern Ireland." In *Gender and Catastrophe*. Edited by Ronit Lentin. London and New York: Zed Books, 1998.

Dublin Abortion Information Campaign flyer, 1992. NIWRM archive.

Dudgeon, Jeffrey. "Background notes in relation to anti-gay legislation in Northern Ireland: Notes prepared in relation to the case, Dudgeon v. United Kingdom to appear at the European Court of Human Rights, 23 April 1981." Dudgeon archive, P10212.

———. "NCCL press statement (Background), European Commission for Human Rights, Application No. 7525/76 lodged by Jeff Dudgeon against the British Government." October 1981. Dudgeon archive.

———. *Roger Casement: The Black Diaries, with a Study of His Background, Sexuality, and Irish Political Life*. Belfast: Belfast Press, 2002.

Duncan, Nancy. "Renegotiating Gender and Sexuality in Public and Private Spaces." In *BodySpace*. Edited by Nancy Duncan. New York and London: Routledge, 1996.

European Court of Human Rights. *Dudgeon v. United Kingdom:* Before the European Court of Human Rights. From *European Human Rights Reports*, no. 149 (1981): 149–87. Linen Hall Library, Northern Ireland Political Collection, P8950.

Feldman, Allen. *Formations of Violence: The Narrative of the Body and Political Terror in Northern Ireland*. Chicago and London: University of Chicago Press, 1991.

Flynn, Leo. "The Irish Supreme Court and the Constitution of Male Homosexuality." In *Legal Inversions: Lesbians, Gay Men, and the Politics of Law*. Edited by Didi Herman and Carl Stychin. Philadelphia: Temple University Press, 1995.

Foucault, Michel. *Discipline and Punish: The Birth of the Prison*. Trans. Alan Sheridan. New York: Pantheon, 1977; New York: Vintage, 1979

———. *The History of Sexuality*. Vol. 1, *An Introduction*. Trans. Robert Hurley. New York: Pantheon, 1978; New York: Vintage Books, 1990.

Frader, Laura L., and Sonya O. Rose, eds. *Gender and Class in Modern Europe*. Ithaca and London: Cornell University Press, 1996.

Frankel, Glenn. "Abortion Case Touches Nerves across Irish Society." *Washington Post*, 19 February 1992, A4.

Fraser, Nancy. *Unruly Practices: Power, Discourse and Gender in Contemporary Social Theory*. Minneapolis: University of Minnesota Press, 1989.

Frazier, Adrian. "Queering the Irish Renaissance." In *Gender and Sexuality in Modern Ireland*. Edited by Bradley and Valiulis.

"The Gay Rights Campaign Answered." *Protestant Telegraph* (Belfast), 2 May 1981, 10.

Goldberg, Jonathan. *Sodometries: Renaissance Texts, Modern Sexualities*. Stanford: Stanford University Press, 1992.

Gould, Stephen Jay. *The Mismeasure of Man*. Rev. and exp. ed. London: Penguin, 1996.

Gray, Jane. "Gender and Uneven Working-Class Formation in the Irish Linen Industry." In *Gender and Class in Modern Europe*. Edited by Frader and Rose.

Habermas, Jurgen. *The Theory of Communicative Action*. Vol. 2, *Lifeworld and System: A Critique of Functionalist Reason*. Trans. Thomas McCarthy. Boston: Beacon Press, 1987.

Hackett, Claire. "Irish, Queer and Equal." *Left Republican Review* 4 (August 2001): 20–23.

———. "Self-determination: The Republican Feminist Agenda." *Feminist Review* 50 (Summer 1995): 111–16.

Hamer, Emily. *Britannia's Glory: A History of Twentieth-Century Lesbians*. London: Cassell, 1996.

Harkin, Margo. *Hush-A-Bye Baby*. Derry Film & Video Workshop, 1989. Film and script.

Harris, Eoghan. "Facing Down Fudge: Now Ireland Can Look Itself in the Face Again." *Sunday Times* (London), 8 March 1992.

Harrison, Henry. *Parnell Vindicated: The Lifting of the Veil*. New York: Richard R. Smith, 1931.

Hauser, Richard. *The Homosexual Society*. London: Bodley Head, 1962.

Hesketh, Tom. *The Second Partitioning of Ireland? The Abortion Referendum of 1983*. Dun Laoghaire: Brandsma Books, 1990.

Higgins, Patrick. *Heterosexual Dictatorship: Male Homosexuality in Postwar Britain*. London: Fourth Estate, 1996.

Holland, Mary. "A Gay Time in Belfast." *New Statesman*, 11 June 1976.

Honan, Marie. "Traitors and British Spies." Presentation given at the annual meeting of the American Conference for Irish Studies. Albany, N.Y., April 1997.

Hyde, H. Montgomery. *The Other Love: An Historical and Contemporary Survey of Homosexuality in Britain*. London: Heineman, 1970.

Inglis, Brian. *Roger Casement*. London: Hodder & Stoughton, 1973.

Ingram, Attracta. Editorial. *Irish Times* (Dublin), 26 February 1992, 27.

Innes, C. L. *Woman and Nation in Irish Literature and Society*. Athens: University of Georgia Press, 1993.

Ireland, Republic of. *Bunreacht na hÉireann*. Dublin: Government Publications Office [Brunswick Press], 1945; 1997; 2000.

———. *Green Paper on Abortion*. Dublin: Government Publications Office, 1999.
———. *A New Framework for Agreement: A Shared Understanding between the British and Irish Governments to Assist Discussion and Negotiation Involving the Northern Ireland Parties*. Dublin: Cahill, 1994.
———. Supreme Court. *McGee v. the Attorney General* [1974] I. R. 284.
———. Supreme Court. *Norris v. the Attorney General*. [1984] I. R. 36.
Irish Lesbian and Gay Organization. "ILGO and the St. Patrick's Day Parade." New York: ILGO, 1998. Flyer/pamphlet.
———. "Let ILGO March!" Cited from http://www.geocities.com/Broadway/5421/ilgospdfaq.html.
"It's Sodomy Says Paisley." *Irish Press* (Dublin), 21 July 77.
Jameson, Fredric. *The Political Unconscious: Narrative as a Socially Symbolic Act*. Ithaca: Cornell University Press, 1981.
Jeffery-Poulter, Stephen. *Peers, Queers, and Commons: The Struggle for Gay Law Reform from 1950 to the Present*. London and New York: Routledge, 1991.
Jeffreys, Sheila. "Does It Matter If They Did It?" In *Not a Passing Phase: Reclaiming Lesbians in History 1840–1985*. Edited by Lesbian History Group. London: Women's Press, 1989.
Jordan, Ellen. *The Woman's Movement and Women's Employment in Nineteenth Century Britain*. London and New York: Routledge, 1999.
Jordan, Neil. *The Crying Game*. Miramax, 1992. Film.
———. *The Crying Game* (screenplay). In *A Neil Jordan Reader*. London: Vintage, 1993.
Katz, Barbara. *Recreating Motherhood*. New York and London: W. W. Norton, 1989.
Kennedy, Kieran. "Official Secrets, Unauthorized Acts." *Irish Literary Supplement* 17.1 (Spring 1998).
Kirkland, Richard. *Identity Parades: Northern Irish Culture and Dissident Subjects*. Liverpool: Liverpool University Press, 2002.
Lehr, Valerie. *Queer Family Values: Debunking the Myth of the Nuclear Family*. Philadelphia: Temple University Press, 1999.
Levine, June. *A Season of Weddings*. Dublin: New Island Books, 1992.
———. *Sisters: The Personal Story of an Irish Feminist*. Swords, Co. Dublin: Ward River Press, 1985.
Lewis, Gifford. *Eva Gore-Booth and Esther Roper: A Biography*. London: Pandora Press, 1988.
Lloyd, David. *Anomalous States: Irish Writing and the Post-Colonial Moment*. Durham: Duke University Press, 1993.
———. "Nationalisms against the State." In *The Politics of Culture in the Shadow of Capital*. Edited by Lisa Lowe and David Lloyd. Durham and London: Duke University Press, 1997.
Longley, Edna. *The Living Stream: Literature and Revisionism in Ireland*. Newcastle upon Tyne, U.K.: Bloodaxe Books, 1994.
Lucas, Norman. *The Great Spy Ring*. London: Arthur Barker, 1966.
Luddy, Maria. *Women in Ireland, 1800–1918: A Documentary History*. Cork: Cork University Press, 1995.

Mackey, H. O. *Roger Casement: The Secret History of the Forged Diaries.* Dublin: Apollo, 1962.

———. *Roger Casement: The Truth about the Forged Diaries.* Dublin: Fallon, 1966.

MacKinnon, Catharine. *Toward a Feminist Theory of the State.* Cambridge: Harvard University Press, 1989.

MacManus, Seumas. *The Story of the Irish Race.* Old Greenwich, Conn.: Devin-Adair, 1921.

Mahaffey, Vicki. *States of Desire: Wilde, Yeats, Joyce, and the Irish Experiment.* New York and Oxford: Oxford University Press, 1998.

Maloney, William J. *The Forged Casement Diaries.* Dublin: Talbot Press, 1936.

Marcus, David, ed. *Alternative Loves: Irish Gay and Lesbian Stories.* Dublin: Martello Books, 1994.

McCafferty, Nell. *A Woman to Blame: The Kerry Babies Case.* Dublin: Attic Press, 1985.

McCann, Eamonn. "Abortion and the Reality of Life in Modern Ireland." *Belfast Telegraph,* 22 September 1999.

———. *Dear God: The Price of Religion in Ireland.* London: Bookmarks, 1999.

McClenaghan, Brendan. "Invisible Comrades: Gays and Lesbians in the Struggle." *Captive Voice/An Glor Gafa* 3.3 (Winter 1991): 21.

McClintock, Anne. "Family Feuds: Gender, Nationalism and the Family." *Feminist Review* 44 (Summer 1993): 61–80.

———. *Imperial Leather: Race, Gender and Sexuality in the Colonial Contest.* New York and London: Routledge, 1995.

McCormack, W. J. *Roger Casement in Death; or, Haunting the Free State.* Dublin: University College Dublin Press, 2002.

McCrudden, Christopher. *Benchmarks for Change: Mainstreaming Fairness in the Governance of Northern Ireland—A Proposal.* Belfast: Committee on the Administration of Justice, 1998.

McDiarmid, Lucy. "The Posthumous Life of Roger Casement." In *Gender and Sexuality in Modern Ireland.* Edited by Bradley and Valiulis.

McGouran, Sean. "A Gay View on Kincora." *Fortnight* 204 (May 1984): 12.

McLoughlin, Micheal T. "Crystal or Glass? A Review of *Dudgeon v. United Kingdom* on the Fifteenth Anniversary of the Decision." *E-Law: Murdoch University Electronic Journal of Law* 3.4 (December 1996). Archived at http://www.murdoch.edu.au/elaw/issues/v3n4/mclough.html (accessed 18 April 2003).

McVeigh, Robbie. *"It's Part of Life Here . . .": The Security Forces and Harassment in Northern Ireland.* Belfast: Committee on the Administration of Justice, 1994.

Meehan, Paula. "The Statue of the Virgin at Granard Speaks." *The Man Who Was Marked by Winter.* Loughcrew, Co. Meath: Gallery Press, 1991.

———. "Home." *f/m* 1 (Summer 1997): 12 (published by Women's Education, Research and Resource Centre, University College Dublin).

Merriman, Brian. *The Midnight Court.* Trans. Patrick C. Power. Cork and Dublin: Mercier, 1971.

Mitchell, Angus, ed. *The Amazon Journal of Roger Casement.* Dublin: Lilliput Press, 1997.

Moloney, Ed, and Andy Pollak. *Paisley: A Biography.* Swords, Co. Dublin: Poolbeg, 1986.

Moore, Chris. *The Kincora Scandal: Political Cover-Up and Intrigue in Northern Ireland.* Dublin: Marino Books, 1996.

Moran, Leslie J. *The Homosexual(ity) of Law.* London and New York: Routledge, 1996.

Morrison, Danny. *On the Back of the Swallow.* Dublin: Mercier, 1994.

Mulkerns, Helena. "Gay Pride and Prejudice." *Hot Press Magazine* (Dublin), April 1995. Cited from http://www.galway.iol.ie/hotpress/iss05951/gaypride.htm.

Nandy, Ashis. *The Intimate Enemy: Loss and Recovery of Self under Colonialism.* Oxford: Oxford University Press, 1983.

NIGRA News (Belfast: June 1976). NIGRA archive.

Norris, David. Criminal Law (Sexual Offences) Bill 1993, Second Stage Speech, Tuesday, 29 June 1993. In *Lesbian and Gay Visions of Ireland: Towards the Twenty-First Century.* Edited by Íde O'Carroll and Eoin Collins. London and New York: Cassell, 1995.

———. "Human Rights for Homosexuals." Letter to the editor. *Irish Times* (Dublin), 29 June 1998, 11.

Noyes, Alfred. *The Accusing Ghost; or, Justice for Casement.* London: Victor Gollancz, 1957.

Oaks, Laury. "Irishness, Eurocitizens, and Reproductive Rights." In *Reproducing Reproduction: Kinship, Power, and Technological Innovation.* Edited by Sarah Franklin and Helena Ragoné. Philadelphia: University of Pennsylvania Press, 1997.

———. "Irishwomen, Euro-citizens and Redefining Abortion." Paper presented at the New England Regional American Conference for Irish Studies, Westfield, Mass., October 1993.

O'Brien, Edna. *Down by the River.* London: Phoenix, 1996.

———. *The High Road.* New York: Farrar, Straus and Giroux, 1988.

———. *Mother Ireland.* New York: Harcourt Brace Jovanovich, 1976.

———. *A Pagan Place.* St. Paul, Minn.: Graywolf Press, 1984.

O'Connor, Frank. "Guests of the Nation." 1931. Reprinted in *Irish Writing in the Twentieth Century.* Edited by David Pierce. Cork: Cork University Press, 2000.

O'Hagan, Martin. "Row as Gay Provo Killer Comes Out of Closet." *Sunday World* (Dublin), 2 February 1992.

O'Reilly, Emily. *Masterminds of the Right.* Dublin: Attic Press, n.d.

Oxford English Dictionary. Oxford and New York: Oxford University Press, 1996.

Paisley, Rev. Ian. "Miss Valerie Shaw's Big Lie Exploded." *Protestant Telegraph* (Belfast), 6 February 1982, 1, 12.

Patton, Cindy. "Tremble, Hetero Swine!" In *Fear of a Queer Planet.* Edited by Michael Warner. Minneapolis and London: University of Minnesota Press, 1993.

Petchesky, Rosalind Pollack. "Fetal Images: The Power of Visual Culture in the Politics of Reproduction." *Feminist Studies* 13 (Summer 1987): 263–92.

Pettitt, Lance. "Pigs and Provos, Prostitutes and Prejudice: Gay Representation in Irish Film, 1984–1995." In *Sex, Nation and Dissent in Irish Writing*. Edited by Éibhear Walshe. Cork: Cork University Press, 1997.

Purdy, Anthony, and Douglas Sutherland. *Burgess and MacLean*. Garden City, N.Y.: Doubleday, 1963.

QueerSpace. "About QueerSpace," 2002. Available at http://www.cara-friend .org.uk/queerspace/aboutqs.htm.

———. "QueerSpace Mission Statement," 1998. Flyer. Available at http:// queerspace.org.uk/; select "About QueerSpace" and then "Mission" (accessed 28 April 2003).

———. "QueerSpace Policy," 1998. Cited from http://www.geocities.com/ WestHollywood/Heights/7124/about.html.

———. "Welcome to QueerSpace, Belfast." Available at http://queerspace .org.uk/ (accessed 28 April 2003).

"The Raced Celt: 1840–1890; An Electronic Primary Text Sourcebook." Archived at http://www.people.virginia.edu/~dnp5c/Victorian/ (accessed 18 April 2003).

"Radio 4—On Paisley." *Protestant Telegraph* (Belfast), 17 December 1978, 7.

Reid, B. L. *The Lives of Roger Casement*. New Haven and London: Yale University Press, 1976.

Riddick, Ruth. "The Right to Choose: Questions of Feminist Morality." 1990. Reprinted in *A Dozen Lips*. Dublin: Attic Press, 1994.

Robbins, Bruce, ed. *The Phantom Public Sphere*. Minneapolis: University of Minnesota Press, 1993.

Rose, Kieran. *Diverse Communities: The Evolution of Lesbian and Gay Politics in Ireland*. *Undercurrents* pamphlet series. Cork: Cork University Press, 1994.

Rothman, Barbara Katz. "Fetal Images: The Power of Visual Culture in the Politics of Reproduction." *Feminist Studies* 13 (Summer 1987).

———. *Recreating Motherhood: Ideology and Technology in a Patriarchal Society*. New York and London: W. W. Norton, 1989.

———. *The Tentative Pregnancy: Prenatal Diagnosis and the Future of Motherhood*. New York: Viking, 1986.

Sales, Rosemary. *Women Divided: Gender, Religion, and Politics in Northern Ireland*. London: Routledge, 1997.

Sawyer, Roger, ed. *Roger Casement's Diaries: 1910: The Black and the White*. London: Pimlico, 1997.

———. *Casement: The Flawed Hero*. London: Routledge, 1984.

Sedgwick, Eve Kosofsky. *Epistemology of the Closet*. Berkeley: University of California Press, 1990.

Segal, Lynne. *Slow Motion: Changing Masculinities, Changing Men*. London: Virago, 1997.

Sharrock, David, and Mark Devenport. *Man of Peace, Man of War: The Unauthorized Biography of Gerry Adams*. London: Macmillan/Pan, 1998.

Sinfield, Alan. *The Wilde Century: Effeminacy, Oscar Wilde, and the Queer Movement*. New York: Columbia University Press, 1994.

Sinn Féin. Ard Fheis debates, 1986. Linen Hall Library, Northern Ireland Political collection, PV 333. Videotape.

———. *Women in Ireland: Sinn Féin Update Policy Document.* Dublin: Sinn Féin, March 1999.

———. *The Politics of Revolution (main speeches and debates 1986 Sinn Féin Ard-Fheis).* Belfast and Dublin: Republican Publications, 1986.

Smyth, Ailbhe. *The Abortion Papers: Ireland.* Dublin: Attic Press, 1992.

———. "'And Nobody Was Any the Wiser': Irish Abortion Rights and the European Union." In *Sexual Politics and the New European Union: The New Feminist Challenge.* Edited by Amy Elman. New York: Berghahn Books, 1996.

———. "Declining Identities." *Critical Survey* 8.2 (1996). Reprinted in *Irish Writing in the Twentieth Century.* Edited by David Pierce. Cork: Cork University Press, 2000.

———. Foreword to *Alternative Loves: Irish Gay and Lesbian Stories.* Edited by David Marcus.

Society for the Protection of Unborn Children. "Threatened by a Human Rights Body/Value Your Voice—Value Your Vote." N.p.: Society for the Protection of Unborn Children, ca. 1990s. Pamphlet.

———. *A Way of Life: Affirming a Pro-Life Culture in Northern Ireland.* 2nd ed. N.p.: Society for the Protection of Unborn Children, March 2002. Archived at http://www.spuc.org.uk/ (accessed 18 April 2003).

Sofia, Zoe. "Exterminating Fetuses: Abortion, Disarmament, and the Sexo-Semiotics of Extraterrestrialism." *Diacritics* 14 (1984): 47–59.

Speth, Carola. "QueerSpace." *Women's News* (Belfast), February 1998, 13.

Squier, Susan. "Fetal Voices: Speaking for the Margins Within." *Tulsa Studies in Women's Literature* 10 (1991): 17–30.

Stallybrass, Peter, and Ann Rosalind Jones. "Dismantling Irena: The Sexualizing of Ireland in Early Modern England." In *Nationalisms and Sexualities.* Edited by Andrew Parker, Mary Russo, Doris Summer, and Patricia Yeager. New York and London: Routledge, 1992.

Stasso, Sally, and Anne Stott. *Rock the Sham.* New York, 1996. Video documentary.

Steinman, Michael. *Yeats's Heroic Figures: Wilde, Parnell, Swift, Casement.* Albany: State University of New York Press, 1984.

Strang, Susan. "Abortion: Whose Body Is It Anyway?" *Women's News* (Belfast) 74 (June/July 1995): 7.

Stychin, Carl F. *A Nation by Rights: National Cultures, Sexual Identity Politics, and the Discourse of Rights.* Philadelphia: Temple University Press, 1998.

Sullivan, A. M. *The Last Serjeant: The Memories of Serjeant A. M. Sullivan, Q. C.* London: Macdonald, 1952.

Sutherland, Douglas. *The Fourth Man: The Story of Blunt, Philby, Burgess and Maclean.* London: Secker & Warburg, 1980.

"Towards Sodom." *Protestant Telegraph* (Belfast), 14 October 1977, 7.

Turner, Martyn. "17 February 1992." *Irish Times* (Dublin), 18 February 1992. Political cartoon.

United Kingdom. *The Belfast Agreement: An Agreement Reached at the Multi-Party Talks on Northern Ireland.* Presented to Parliament by the Secretary of State for Northern Ireland by Command of Her Majesty. London: Her Majesty's Stationery Office, April 1998.

———. *Draft Homosexual Offenses (Northern Ireland) Order 1978.* Belfast: Her Majesty's Stationery Office, 1978.
———. "Observations of the United Kingdom on the Merits of Application No. 7525/76 Lodged by Jeffrey Dudgeon," March 1979. Dudgeon archive.
———. Parliament. House of Commons. *Parliamentary Debates (Hansard), House of Commons Official Report,* vols. 724, 748–49. London: Her Majesty's Stationery Office, 1966–67.
———. Parliament. House of Lords. *Parliamentary Debates (Hansard), House of Lords Official Report,* vols. 266, 284. London: Her Majesty's Stationery Office, 1965, 1967.
———. Standing Advisory Commission on Human Rights. *Report on the Law in Northern Ireland Relating to Divorce and Homosexuality.* London: Her Majesty's Stationery Office, 1977.
———. Standing Advisory Commission on Human Rights. *Sixth Report of the Standing Advisory Commission on Human Rights: Annual Report for 1979–80.* London: Her Majesty's Stationery Office, 5 March 1981.
———. Wolfenden Committee. *Report of the Committee on Homosexual Offences and Prostitution.* London: Her Majesty's Stationery Office, September 1957.
United States. Court of Appeals for the Second Circuit. *The Irish Lesbian and Gay Organization v. Giuliani, et al.* Docket No. 97-7064, 1997–98. Archived at http://csmail.law.pace.edu/lawlib/legal/us-legal/judiciary/second-circuit/test3/97-7064a.opn.html and http://csmail.law.pace.edu/lawlib/legal/us-legal/judiciary/second-circuit/test3/97-7064b.opn.html.
Valente, Joseph. "The Myth of Sovereignty: Gender in the Literature of Irish Nationalism." *English Literary History* 61.10 (1994): 189–210.
Ward, Margaret. *Unmanageable Revolutionaries: Women and Irish Nationalism.* London: Pluto Press, 1983.
Warner, Michael, ed. *Fear of a Queer Planet: Queer Politics and Social Theory.* Minneapolis and London: University of Minnesota Press, 1993.
Weber, Max. "Politics as a Vocation." In *From Max Weber.* Edited by H. H. Geth and C. W. Mills. London: RKP, 1970.
Weeks, Jeffrey. *Coming Out: Homosexual Politics in Britain, from the Nineteenth Century to the Present.* London, Melbourne, and New York: Quartet Books, 1977.
West, Rebecca. *The New Meaning of Treason.* New York: Viking Press, 1964.
———. *The Vassall Affair.* London: Sunday Telegraph, 1963.
Westwood, Gordon. *A Minority: A Report on the Life of the Male Homosexual in Great Britain.* London: Longmans, 1960.
White, Chris, ed. *Nineteenth-Century Writings on Homosexuality: A Sourcebook.* London and New York: Routledge, 1999.
Wittig, Monique. "One Is Not Born a Woman." In *The Lesbian and Gay Studies Reader.* Edited by Henry Abelove, Michèle Aina Barale, and David M. Halperin. New York: Routledge, 1993.
Yeats, William Butler. *The Letters of W. B. Yeats.* Edited by Allan Wade. London: Rupert Hart-Davis, 1954.
———. *The Variorum Edition of the Plays of W. B. Yeats.* Edited by Russell K. Alspach. New York: Macmillan, 1966.

————. *The Variorum Edition of the Poems of W. B. Yeats.* Edited by Peter Allt and Russell K. Alspach. New York: Macmillan, 1957.

Yuval-Davis, Nira. *Gender and Nation.* London: Sage Publications, 1997.

Zwicker, Heather. "Gendered Troubles: Refiguring 'Woman' in Northern Ireland." *Genders* 19 (1994): 198–222.

Index

Irish Studies in Literature and Culture

www.ingramcontent.com/pod-product-compliance
Lightning Source LLC
Chambersburg PA
CBHW050222270326
41914CB00003BA/527